# MEDICAL RESEARCH ESSENTIALS

W0114172

**Notice**

Medicine is an ever-changing science. As new research and clinical experience broaden our knowledge, changes in treatment and drug therapy are required. The authors and the publisher of this work have checked with sources believed to be reliable in their efforts to provide information that is complete and generally in accord with the standards accepted at the time of publication. However, in view of the possibility of human error or changes in medical sciences, neither the authors nor the publisher nor any other party who has been involved in the preparation or publication of this work warrants that the information contained herein is in every respect accurate or complete, and they disclaim all responsibility for any errors or omissions or for the results obtained from use of the information contained in this work. Readers are encouraged to confirm the information contained herein with other sources. For example and in particular, readers are advised to check the product information sheet included in the package of each drug they plan to administer to be certain that the information contained in this work is accurate and that changes have not been made in the recommended dose or in the contraindications for administration. This recommendation is of particular importance in connection with new or infrequently used drugs.

# MEDICAL RESEARCH ESSENTIALS

Rania Esteitie, MD, BS in Biology
Resident Physician
Department of Internal Medicine
St. Elizabeth's Medical Center
Boston, Massachusetts

Formerly:
Post-Doctoral Research Fellow and Resident Physician
Department of Internal Medicine
Georgetown University Hospital
Washington, District of Columbia

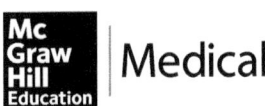
Medical

New York / Chicago / San Francisco / Athens / London / Madrid
Mexico City / Milan / New Delhi / Singapore / Sydney / Toronto

Medical Research Essentials

Copyright © 2014 by McGraw-Hill Education. All rights reserved. Printed in the United States of America. Except as permitted under the United States Copyright Act of 1976, no part of this publication may be reproduced or distributed in any form or by any means, or stored in a data base or retrieval system, without the prior written permission of the publisher.

1 2 3 4 5 6 7 8 9 0   DOC/DOC   18  17  16  15  14  13

ISBN 978-0-07-178164-0
MHID 0-07-178164-1

This book was set in Sabon by Thomson Digital.
The editors were Catherine A. Johnson and Regina Y. Brown.
The production supervisor was Richard Ruzycka.
Project management was provided by Shaminder Pal Singh, Thomson Digital.
RR Donnelley was printer and binder.

This book is printed on acid-free paper.

Cataloging-in-Publication data for this title is on file with the Library of Congress.

McGraw-Hill Education books are available at special quantity discounts to use as premiums and sales promotions, or for use in corporate training programs. To contact a representative please visit the Contact Us pages at www.mhprofessional.com.

# Dedication

*To my loving husband Yousef: for making my life "significantly" better just by being in it. To my baby Talia: may this book be the first step toward a lifetime of knowledge.*

*To my incredible family: where the heart knows no distance.*
*Mom: for your incredible undying support.*
*Dad: the most intelligent person I know.*
*My incredible sisters (Farah and Yasmine): who taught me the meaning of unconditional love and brewed in me the spirit of laughter.*

# CONTENTS

# PREFACE

Evidence-based medicine (EBM) has become a vital aspect in today's practice of medicine. The plethora of new medical knowledge, research, and innovative technology begets constant referral to the medical literature for the most up-to-date advances. Most of today's recommendations and guidelines for medical treatment and diagnosis stem from research. Therefore, to apply them in one's practice, let alone practice it, one must fully first understand them.

The objective of this book is to guide and direct medical students and residents interested in performing research projects during their medical education. It serves as a mini-mentor in and of itself with numerous tips and guidelines as to what medical students and residents need to know in order to complete a research project in a limited amount of time. It is targeted for use in all medical institutions practicing EBM as a starter kit for those interested in performing a research project. Topics that are included focus on the types of research studies that are amenable to completion based on a specific time frame, how to read the medical literature, how to organize and analyze data, and how to design your own study, as well as an easy guide to the understanding and implementation of medical statistics.

The topic is depicted in a practical and conceptual approach. This manual is based on a survey I conducted asking residents and students what would have made it easier for them to conduct research during their training. The main objective is to save them time from searching endless websites for an approach to research and having everything combined into one small handbook. This in no means is a complicated, verbose piece of medical literature. Rather, it contains numerous flowcharts, algorithms, diagrams, and tables that will aid in illustrating my point as opposed to a lot of writing.

The main audience for this book is medical students and residents. Numerous medical institutions are now advocating a more evidence-based medical approach to their medical education and are therefore placing heavy emphasis on performing research during their training years. Because time is of the essence, this manual combines everything they need to know about research, including reading it, understanding it, and ultimately performing it, so that they are able to complete their requirements for training.

I would like to acknowledge my research mentors at The University of Chicago and National Institutes of Health, without whom I would have never had all the incredible learning opportunities that I was lucky enough to have encountered. Dr. Baroody, Dr. Pinto, and Dr. Togias—thank you for showing me how much I didn't know about research that inspired me to write this book!

# ACKNOWLEDGMENTS

I would like to thank Fahad Barakat: my understanding of statistics would have been next to nil if it wasn't for his help.

# MEDICAL
# RESEARCH
# ESSENTIALS

# INTRODUCTION

## WHY EVIDENCE-BASED MEDICINE?

*Evidence-based medicine is the conscientious, explicit, and judicious use of the best current evidence in making decisions about the care of individual patients.*
—David L. Sackett, et al., BMJ. 1996;312:71

Evidence-based medicine (EBM) is an ongoing and burgeoning field that has now become the norm in today's practice of medicine. It is defined as the union of individual clinical expertise with the most current research evidence and patient values (Fig. 1.1).[1] It involves a systematic approach to clinical problems aimed at identifying strategies that work and eliminating those that do not work, are harmful, or are proven to be not beneficial based on research evidence.[2] EBM promotes critical thinking. It demands that the effectiveness of clinical interventions, the accuracy and precision of diagnostic tests, and the power of prognostic markers be scrutinized and their usefulness proven. It requires clinicians to be open minded and look for and try new methods that are scientifically proven to be effective and to discard methods shown to be ineffective or harmful. Given the heavy emphasis on EBM, it is therefore critical to understand the elements of this in order to use it in practice.

The "evidence" points to what is the best practice available today, and that may change within days to years. Applying the knowledge gained from large clinical trials to patient care promotes consistency of treatment and optimal outcomes, helps establish national standards of patient care, and sets criteria to measure and reward performance-based medical practice.[3] Implementing the principles of EBM, which rely on the rules of evidence and research, requires a commitment from

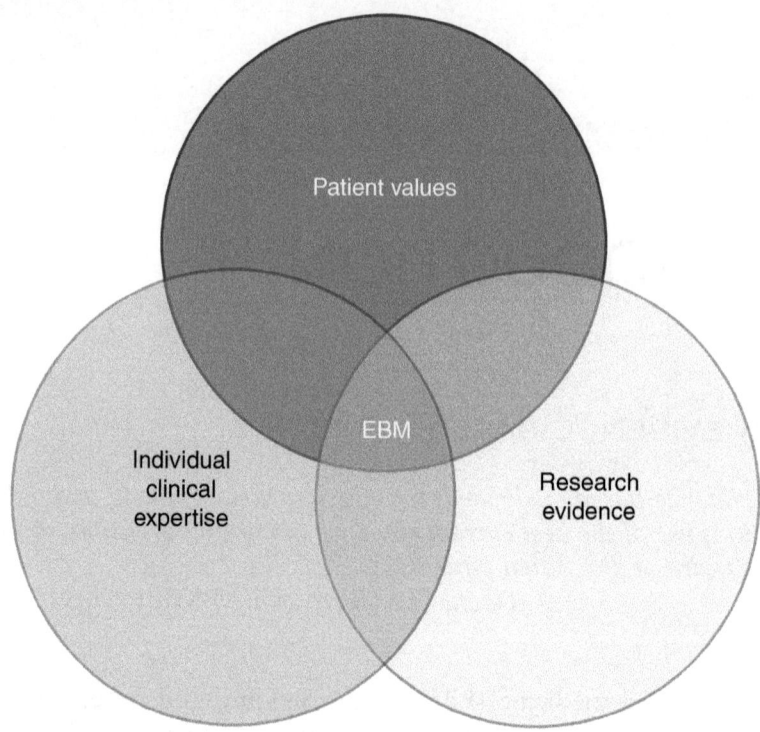

**FIGURE 1.1** Evidence-based medicine (EBM) Venn diagram. EBM is defined as the union of individual clinical expertise with the most current research evidence and patient values.

medical schools, local health and medical licensing departments, physicians, pharmacists, professional associations, and managed care organizations. This kind of commitment can come in various forms such as emphasis on research projects, journal clubs, didactics, team rounds, and finally individualized assessments.

The elements of EBM are summarized in five simple steps:

1. Asking a focused question: One of the most difficult steps in practicing medicine in general is translating a patient clinical problem into a well-structured question. Many questions can arise when confronted with a clinical scenario. However, one must develop skills to convert this information into a focused clinical question that is relevant to the problem at hand. The next step is how to phrase that question in order to facilitate the search. A useful framework was developed by Sackett et al[1] in which they proposed that a good clinical question should address four main elements abbreviated as PICO: the patient or population at hand (P), the intervention or exposure (I),

the comparison (C), and the clinical outcomes (O) that are associated with it. All these elements comprise the PICO method for asking a clinical question that proves to be helpful in not only asking a clinical question but also appraising the literature. An additional element can be added to this framework to account for time (T). An example of implanting this method is as follows:

Imagine that a 50-year-old male patient with no risk factors comes to see you in your clinic and asks you whether he should take aspirin to prevent cardiovascular disease. Following the PICOT method:

P: A healthy adult

I: Aspirin

C: No aspirin

O: Cardiovascular disease

T: In 5 years

Therefore, the question you should ask would be: In an otherwise healthy man with no risk factors or medical conditions, what is the benefit of taking aspirin versus no aspirin in preventing cardiovascular disease in 5 years? This question, now focused, can be placed in the EBM paradigm in order to provide the patient with the best care. The PICOT method is described in detail in Chapter 2.

2. Finding the evidence behind that question: Typically, this is done by searching the literature by way of national databases, guidelines, and journal articles. Combining the current accepted and tested parameters with one's experience and expertise is the most effective method for obtaining the best approach for one's patients. The ability to search these databases effectively is yet an important aspect of EBM, since it is important to be able to extract the relevant pieces of data that are pertinent to your question. Basic search principles include:

a. Convert a clinical problem into a question (achieved in the first step in EBM).

b. Generate appropriate keywords.

c. Choose a bibliographic database. There are numerous online databases, including PubMed, MEDLINE, EMBASE, and Cochrane. The Cochrane library includes a database of systematic reviews, controlled trials, and abstracts, which is updated quarterly by an international initiative and available via the internet.

d. Conduct the search. At the basic level, an efficient method is to combine individual words or terms using the Boolean operators "AND" and "OR".[4] If you are combining two terms, AND allows only articles containing both terms to be retrieved, and OR allows articles containing either term to be retrieved. Sometimes results of a search can retrieve an innumerable amount of hits, which can be further queried based on one's own preferences such as time period (2000–2013) and types of study (randomized controlled trials only).

3. Appraising the evidence: Although there is a wealth of research articles available, the quality of these is variable. After the appropriate information and evidence have been compiled, the next step is to test it for validity, applicability, and clinical relevance. This is vital because each clinical scenario is different and unique and requires delicate fine-tuning to make sure that it is applicable and sound for that clinical scenario and especially for that patient's own wishes. Several tools for appraising research articles are available, for example the tools developed by the Critical Appraisal Skills Programme (CASP), Oxford, United Kingdom. These include tools for appraising randomized controlled trials, systematic reviews, case-control studies, and cohort studies (this is also discussed further in Chapter 2).[5] Additional ways to appraise the evidence also take the form of "levels of evidence" and "grading the strength of recommendations."

4. Applying the evidence: The first step is to determine whether this evidence can be applied in clinical practice. Next one should apply their own expertise to the pertinent evidence and guide the patient in making an informed decision using the available data. Research evidence includes systematic observations from the laboratory, preliminary pathophysiological studies, and more advanced applied clinical research, such as randomized controlled trials.[6] This decision should also take into account costs and the availability of that particular treatment in practice.

5. Evaluating performance: After the decision has been made, the last and final step rests in evaluating whether the decision was the most appropriate (Fig. 1.2).

Evidence-based medicine therefore aids in improving the quality of care, patient access, treatment outcomes, appropriateness of care, efficiency and effectiveness, and cost containment by improving the cost-to-benefit ratio. Therefore, it is essential for all clinicians to develop these skills.

Staying "current" and up to date on current recommendations and guidelines remains a challenge. It is especially not easy for medical students and residents, given their long work hours and study schedule, to find time to become a part of this paradigm. Although a majority of

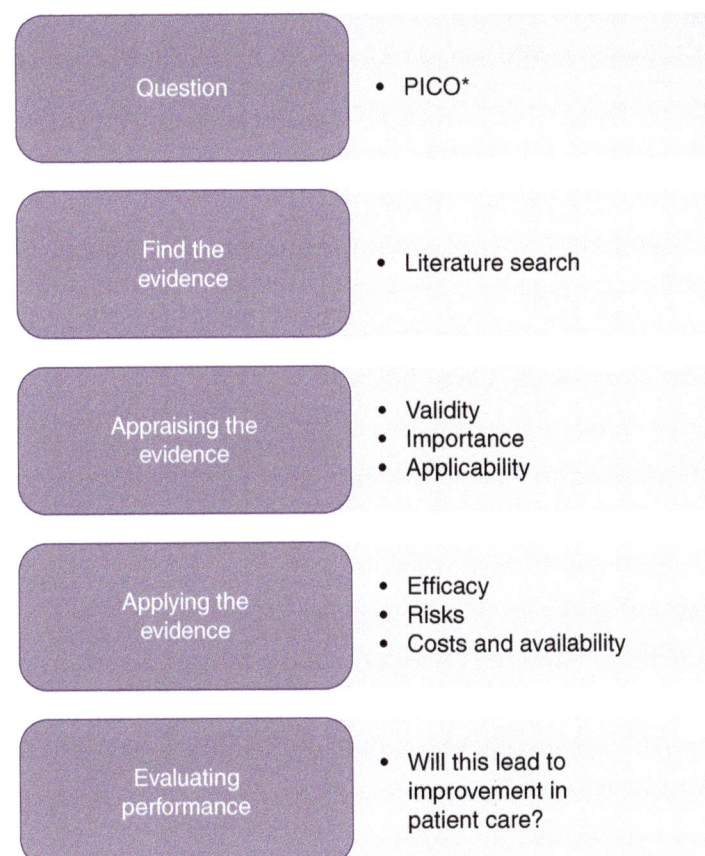

**FIGURE 1.2** Approach to evidence-based medicine (EBM). EBM involves five main steps: (1) asking a focused question through the PICO method (*explained in detail in Chapter 2); (2) finding the evidence behind that question via a literature search; (3) appraising the evidence and testing it for validity, applicability, and clinical relevance; (4) applying the evidence in the form of making a decision; and (5) evaluating performance to patient care.

programs recently have focused on EBM as part of research, it remains a field heavily emphasized primarily in competitive programs.

The purpose of this book is to provide a research guide to medical students and residents to help them understand the elements of research in a practical way and to aid them in translating their own questions and clinical problems into solid research projects. Training physicians who are adept at evaluating the literature with an EBM perspective would allow for providing the best medical care at the lowest cost and achieving optimal outcomes.

References

1. Sackett DL, Rosenberg WM, Gray JA, Haynes RB, Richardson WS. Evidence based medicine: what it is and what it isn't. *BMJ*. 1996;312:71.

2. Akobeng AK. Principles of evidence based medicine. *Arch Dis Child*. 2005;90: 837-840.

3. Lewis SJ, Orland BI. The importance and impact of evidence-based medicine. *J Manag Care Pharm*. 2004;10(5 Suppl A):S3-S5.

4. Craig JV, Smyth RL. *The Evidence-Based Manual for Nurses*. London: Churchill Livingstone; 2002.

5. Critical Appraisal Skills Programme. Appraisal Tools. http://www.casp-uk.net/find-appraise-act/appraising-the-evidence/

6. Haynes RB, Devereaux PJ, Guyatt GH. Clinical expertise in the era of evidence-based medicine and patient choice. *Evid Based Med*. 2002;7:36-38.

# HOW TO CLASSIFY
# RESEARCH STUDIES

The quality and reliability of a study are influenced by the type of study design selected.[1] This selection is determined by the specific question to be answered and aids in depicting the usefulness of a study and the ease of its interpretation. In principle, medical research is classified into primary and secondary research. Primary Research: involves direct participation of the authors and can be classified into interventional (or experimental) and noninterventional (or observational) studies (Fig. 2.1). Secondary research: summarizes one or more primary or secondary sources (in the form of reviews or meta-analyses), usually to provide an overview of a medical topic. These are typically performed in primary research studies.

The research question at hand determines which research study would be the best in answering the question. For example, to measure causality, the best study used would be a randomized controlled trial (RCT) as opposed to a cross-sectional study that cannot measure causality. To study rare outcomes, case-control studies are typically the best ones used. In the interest of time and money, cross-sectional studies, case series, and meta-analysis tend to be the most preferred methods (Table 2.1).[2,3]

The choice of study type also depends on the tools that are available at the time. In a case-control study, investigators start with diseased and control subjects and go back in time to determine whether exposure has occurred. In a retrospective cohort, investigators start with the disease and go back in time to determine whether or not exposure was present. In a prospective cohort, investigators start with exposed and nonexposed groups and determine whether the disease later occurs (Fig. 2.2).

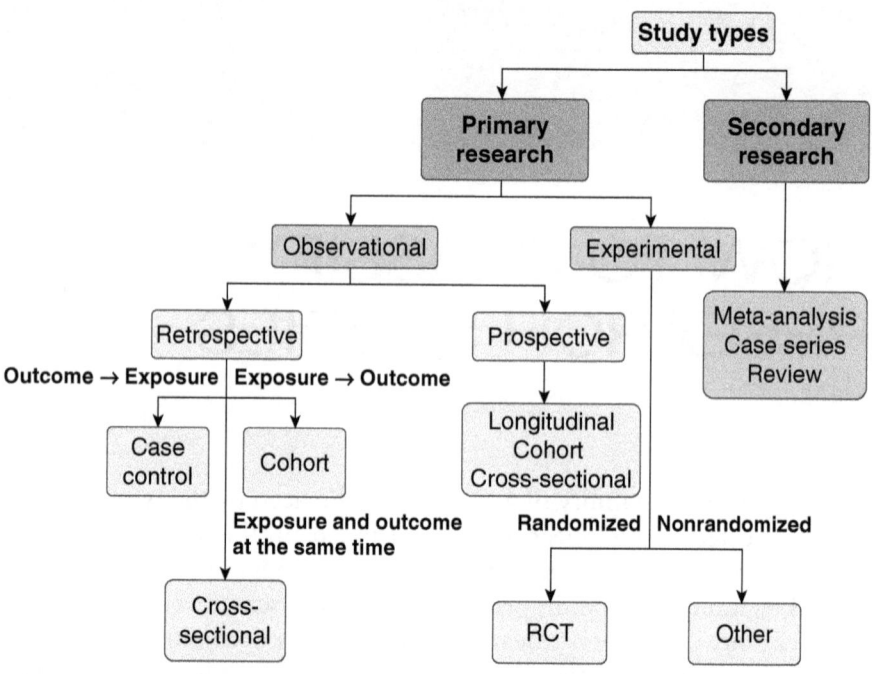

**FIGURE 2.1** Summary of study types. Research can be categorized into primary (observational vs. experimental) or secondary (meta-analysis, case series). Further classification depends on how and when data are collected and whether randomization took place.

## INTERVENTIONAL AND EXPERIMENTAL STUDIES

The aim of an interventional clinical study is to compare treatment procedures within a patient population, which should exhibit as few as possible internal differences apart from the treatment. This is to be achieved by appropriate measures, particularly by random allocation of the patients to the groups, thus avoiding bias in the result. International recommendations for the reporting of randomized clinical studies can be found in the CONSORT (Consolidated Standards of Reporting Trials) statement (www.consort-statement.org).[4]

Blinding is another suitable method to avoid bias. A distinction is made between single and double blinding. With single blinding, the patient is unaware of which treatment he or she is receiving. With double blinding, neither the patient nor the investigator knows which treatment is planned. Thus, double blinding ensures that the patient or therapy groups are both handled and observed in the same manner.

Another method of designs interventional studies is by using a parallel study design. A parallel study is a type of clinical study in which

**TABLE 2.1** Advantages and Disadvantages of the Different Research Study Designs.

| Type | Advantages | Disadvantages | Statistics |
|------|-----------|---------------|------------|
| Randomized controlled trial | Measure causality, controls unmeasured confounders | Expensive, takes time, lost to follow-up | |
| Cohort (prospective or retrospective) | Some evidence of causality, multiple outcomes of a single exposure | Expensive, inefficient for rare outcomes, loss to follow-up, requires long follow-up or large population, cannot control unmeasured confounders | Incidence, RR, OR |
| Case control | Rare outcomes, work backwards (outcome → exposure), can generate hypothesis (multiple RF explored) | No causality, selection bias, recall bias, no incidence or prevalence | OR |
| Cross-sectional | Fast, inexpensive, no loss to follow-up, associations can be made | Cannot study causality, cannot study rare outcomes | Prevalence |
| Meta-analysis | Greater statistical power, confirmatory data analysis<br>Greater ability to extrapolate to general population affected<br>Considered an evidence-based resource | Difficult and time-consuming to identify appropriate studies<br>Not all studies provide adequate data for inclusion and analysis<br>Requires advanced statistical techniques<br>Heterogeneity of study populations | |
| Case series | Describes trends, cheap, easy | | |

OR, odds ratio; RF, risk factors; RR, relative risk.

two groups of treatments, A and B, are given so that one group receives only A while another group receives only B. This is unlike a crossover study in which at first one group receives treatment A later followed by treatment B while the other group receives treatment B followed by treatment A (Table 2.2).

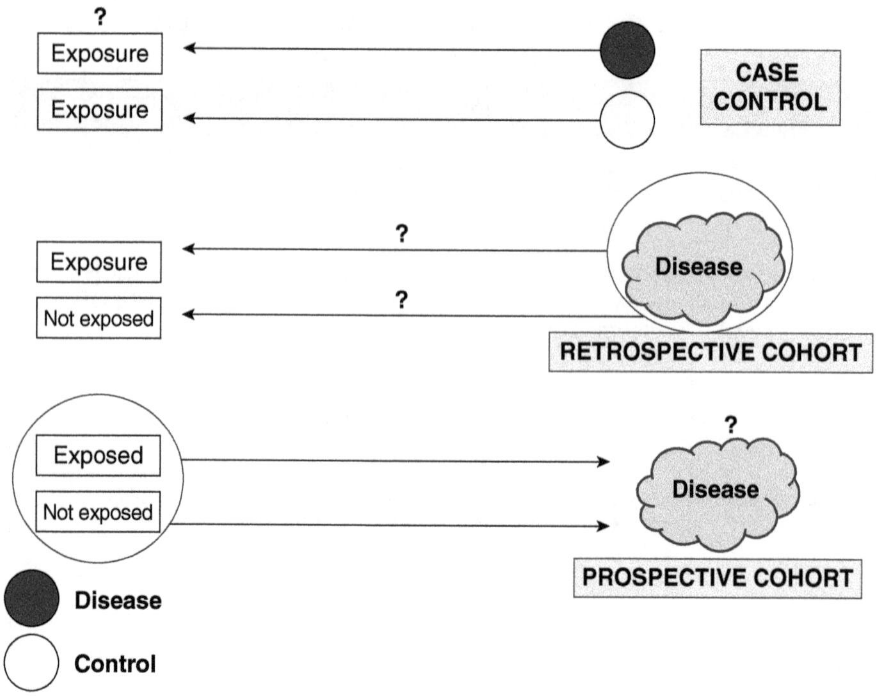

FIGURE 2.2 Case-control versus cohort studies. In a case-control study, investigators start with diseased and control subjects and go back in time to determine whether exposure has occurred. In a retrospective cohort, investigators start with the disease and go back in time to determine whether or not exposure was present. In a prospective cohort, the investigators start with exposed and nonexposed groups and determine whether the disease later occurs.

Typically used in therapeutic trials when two treatments cannot be made identical. Double-dummy studies are typically used in therapeutic trials when two treatments cannot be made identical. This consists of having Drug A and its indistinguishable Placebo A and Drug B with its own indistinguishable Placebo B. Patients then take either Treatment A (Active Drug A and placebo B) or Treatment B (Active Drug B and placebo A) (Fig. 2.3).

## OBSERVATIONAL STUDIES

Observational epidemiologic studies can be further subdivided into cohort studies (follow-up studies), case-control studies, and cross-sectional studies (prevalence studies). Studies with only descriptive evaluation are restricted to a simple depiction of the frequency (incidence and prevalence) and distribution of a disease within a population.

**TABLE 2.2** Research Methodological Designs.

| Study Design | Description |
|---|---|
| Parallel comparison | Each group receives a different treatment with both groups being entered at the same time. Results are analyzed by comparing groups. |
| Single blind | Only subjects are blinded to the treatment or intervention they receive. |
| Double blind | Both subjects and investigators are blind to the treatment or intervention they receive. |
| Cross-over | Each subject receives the intervention, and the control treatments (in random order) are often separated by a washout period. |
| Double dummy | Double dummy is a method of blinding where both treatment groups may receive placebo. One group may receive Treatment A and the placebo of Treatment B; the other group would receive Treatment B and the placebo of Treatment A. |
| Open label | A research trial in which in which both the researchers and participants know which treatment is being administered |

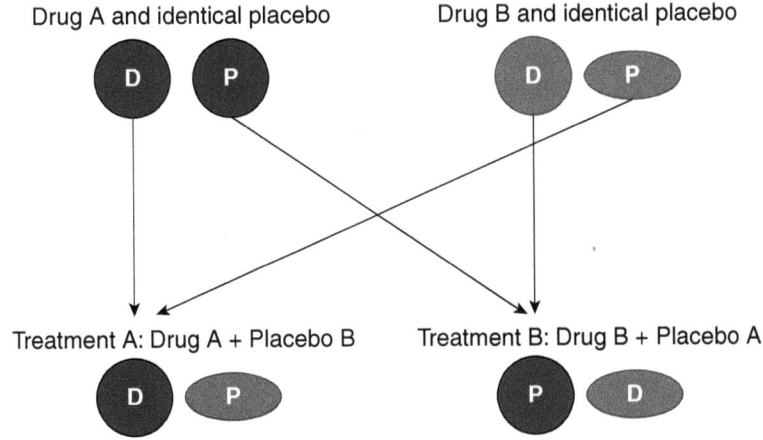

**FIGURE 2.3** Double-dummy trial. This type of trial is typically used in therapeutic trials when two treatments cannot be made identical. This consists of having Drug A and its indistinguishable Placebo A and Drug B with its indistinguishable Placebo B. Patients then take either Treatment A (Active Drug A and placebo B) or Treatment B (Active Drug B and placebo A).

Cohort studies involve the observation of two healthy groups of subjects over time. One group is exposed to a specific substance, and the other is not exposed. Then the frequency of a specific outcome is recorded prospectively. The relative risk (quotient of the incidence rates) is a very important statistical parameter that can be calculated in cohort studies. Cohort studies are well suited for detecting causal connections between exposure and the development of disease but often demand a great deal of time, organization, and money.[5]

## TESTING THESE STUDIES

The aim of evidence-based medicine (EBM) is to provide the best answer to a clinical question.[6] One way to get evidence is to search the literature to identify relevant articles and evaluate (or critically appraise) the quality of the articles.[7] Although an innumerable amount of literature exists today, it would be impossible to get through it all in a timely manner. Levels of evidence are one way to sift through all this literature. The principle behind levels of evidence is that all articles constitute evidence but some are more persuasive through virtue of their study design. The deliberations of evidence-based analysis are usually summarized as recommendations, graded by the number and quality of studies[8] (Table 2.3).

### Levels of Evidence

Levels of evidence is a method used in EBM to determine the clinical value of a study. The highest and most trustworthy level, level 1 evidence tends to arise from RCTs or meta-analyses of RCT. Level 2 evidence stems from prospective comparative studies, meta-analysis of level 2 studies, or level 1 studies with inconsistent results. Level 3 evidence

**TABLE 2.3** Levels of Evidence and Grades of Recommendation.

| Grade of Recommendation | Level of Evidence | Interventions |
| --- | --- | --- |
| A | 1a | Systemic review of RCTs |
|   | 1b | Individual RCT |
| B | 2a | Systematic review of cohort studies |
|   | 2b | Individual cohort study |
|   | 3a | Systematic review of case-control studies |
|   | 3b | Individual case-control study |
| C | 4 | Case series |
| D | 5 | Expert opinion or bench research |

describes data from retrospective cohort studies, or case-control studies, or meta-analysis of level 3 studies (observational studies with controls). Level 4 evidence describes data from case series (observational studies without controls). Finally, the poorest level of evidence, level 5, arises from case reports, expert opinions, and personal observations.

## Grades

There are four grades of recommendation: A, B, C, and D. Treatments that receive an A are supported by good evidence (level I studies with consistent finding) for or against recommending intervention. Treatments that receive a B are supported by fair evidence (level II or III studies or extrapolations from level 1 studies). C-graded treatments have conflicting or poor-quality evidence (level IV or extrapolations from level II or III studies) not allowing a recommendation for or against intervention. Treatments that receive a D do not have sufficient evidence to make a recommendation and are typically derived from level V evidence or inconsistent or inconclusive studies of any level.

## References

1. Röhrig B, du Prel JB, Wachtlin D, Blettner M. Types of study in medical research. *Dtsch Arztebl Int.* 2009;106(15):262-268.
2. Fleiss JL. *The Design and Analysis of Clinical Experiments.* New York: John Wiley & Sons; 1986:149-185.
3. Machin D, Campbell MJ. *Design of Studies for Medical Research.* Chichester, UK: Wiley; 2005:1-286.
4. Moher D, Schulz KF, Altman DG; CONSORT GROUP (Consolidated Standards of Reporting Trials). The CONSORT statement: revised recommendations for improving the quality of reports of parallel-group randomized trials. *Ann Intern Med.* 2001;134(8):657-662.
5. Creswell JWl. *Research Design: Qualitative, Quantitative, and Mixed Methods Approaches.* Thousand Oaks, CA: Sage Publications; 2003.
6. Walliman N. *Your Research Project: A Step-by-Step Guide for the First-Time Researcher.* London: Sage Publications; 2001.
7. Altman DG, Gore SM, Gardner MJ, Pocock SJ. Statistical guidelines for contributors to medical journals. *Br Med J (Clin Res Ed).* 1983;286:1489-1493.
8. Guyatt GH, Oxman AD, Vist G, Kunz R, Falck-Ytter Y, Alonso-Coello P, Schünemann HJ, for the GRADE Working Group. Rating quality of evidence and strength of recommendations GRADE: an emerging consensus on rating quality of evidence and strength of recommendations. *BMJ.* 2008;336:924-926.

## Suggested Readings

Sackett DL, Straus SE, Richardson WS, et al. *Evidence-Based Medicine: How to Practice and Teach EBM.* 2nd ed. Edinburgh, Scotland: Churchill Livingstone; 2000:173-177.
Sackett DL. Evidence based medicine: what it is and what it isn't. *Br Med J.* 1996;312: 71-72.

# JOURNAL CLUB

## *How to read and critique an article*

Clinicians have 0.7 to 18.5 questions for every 10 patients they care for.[1,2] However, answers to two-thirds of the questions are either not pursued or pursued but not found.[3,4] Subsequent analyses show that almost all unanswered questions could be answered through improved query formulation and better search.[2] Critical appraisal is a systematic process used to identify the strengths and weaknesses of a research article in order to assess the usefulness and validity of research findings. The most important components of a critical appraisal are an evaluation of the appropriateness of the study design for the research question and a careful assessment of the key methodological features of this design.[5] This draws clinicians to read journal articles that represent the most recent advancements in research and treatment methods in a specific area. Medical institutions recently have focused on adopting and practicing evidence-based medicine.[6,7] One of the ways this is implemented is through journal clubs. These clubs introduce medical personnel to novel advancements in a particular field but also help set the stage for future research endeavors. Because journal clubs are usually an hour long, each person has a limited amount of time to discuss the article. The algorithm below serves to guide and help build the background in dissecting an article.

### APPROACH TO AN ARTICLE

Whether it is journal club or simply just reading a journal article, it is important to approach an article in the same systematic and organized manner. It can become very intimidating, especially if someone does not have a background in the research field. Therefore, one should approach each article in the same manner and keep in mind certain crucial points that are significant in understanding and analyzing any article. The following points coupled with the journal club worksheet provided in this chapter will serve as an introduction and helpful learning tool in understanding how to dissect a research article (Fig. 3.1).

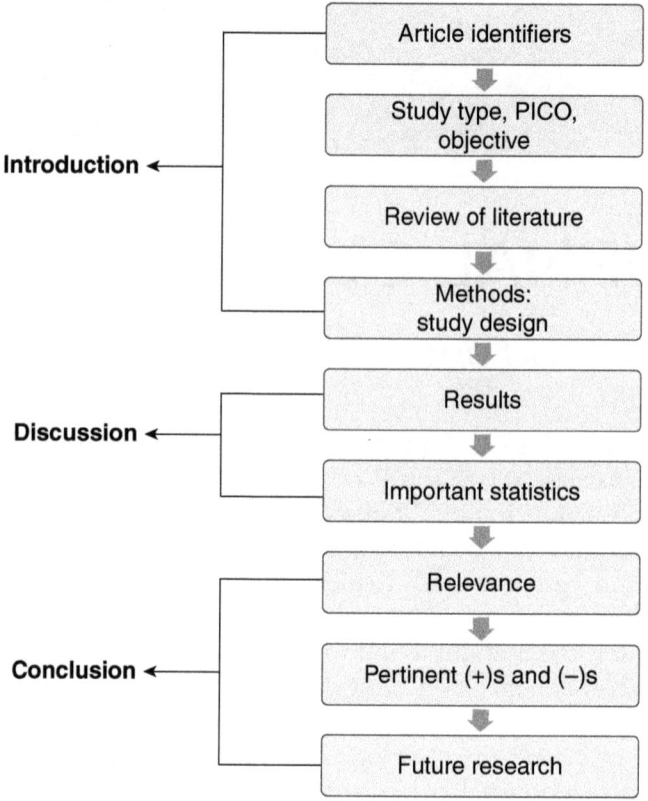

**FIGURE 3.1** The article dissector. This algorithm serves as the basic approach to dissecting an article. The article is divided into three main parts: the introduction, discussion, and conclusion.

## Introduction

In order to dissect a journal article, one should divide it into three main sections: the introduction, discussion, and conclusion. The introduction should further encompass four main elements: article identifiers, study type/PICO(T), a review of the medical literature, and methods.

### Article Identifiers

The beginning of every journal club should start with the main article identifiers, which are the article name, author, journal, and year. This serves as an introduction to the talk that is crucial to the presentation as a whole.

### Study Type

After introducing the article, it is important to state the type of study because this sets the stage for determining the quality, reliability, and

validity of the study as it applies to the clinical domain. This information is significant because it determines the applicability of the study
and accuracy in determining whether its results should be taken into
consideration in real practice and whether their recommendations set
the stage for future development of guidelines.

To recognize the type of study, one should ask three questions:

1. Aim of the study
   a. To simply describe a population → descriptive
   b. To quantify the relationship between factors (PICO applicable) →
      analytic

2. If analytic:
   a. Randomized → randomized controlled trial (RCT)
   b. Nonrandomized → experimental

3. When the outcomes were determined
   a. Some time after the exposure or intervention → prospective cohort
   b. At the same time of the exposure or intervention → cross-sectional
   c. Before the exposure was determined → case-control retrospective
      study (Table 3.1)

## PICO(T)

The adequate (well-constructed) research question allows for the correct
definition of which information (evidence) is needed to solve the clinical
research question.[8,9] In approaching an article, especially in the introduction, one should always keep in mind the PICO(T) algorithm. The
PICO strategy can be used to construct several kinds of research questions, originated from clinical practice, human and material resource
management, the search of symptom assessment instruments, among
others[8,10] (see Fig. 3.2). This includes identifying the type or patients or
population studied coupled with the intervention performed (if any),
the comparison used, the studied outcomes, and the time in which the
study was conducted. Within this paradigm, you would introduce the
objective and aims of the study. This method is easily applied to experimental studies; however, this may be a bit challenging in certain studies.
The PICO(T) method is best used in analytic studies.[11,12] This includes
experimental analytic (RCT or controlled trials) and observational analytic studies (cohorts, cross-sectional, case series). It would therefore be
difficult to apply this method, specifically the intervention aspect of it to
non-analytic studies (systematic reviews/meta-analysis, cross-sectional
surveys). Therefore, it would only be possible to apply the P and O
(patient or population) and outcome.

**TABLE 3.1** Types of Research Studies.

| Study Type | Description |
| --- | --- |
| **Observational** | |
| Cohort | Cohorts are a group of participants with a similar characteristic that are followed through time (either retrospectively or prospectively) to determine which risk factors are associated with that particular characteristic. |
| Case control | A study that compares patients who have a disease or outcome of interest (cases) with patients who do not have the disease or outcome (control participants) and looks back retrospectively to compare how frequently the exposure to a risk factor is present in each group to determine the relationship between the risk factor and the disease. |
| Cross-sectional | Observation of all of a population, or a representative subset, at one specific point in time. They differ from case-control studies in that they aim to provide data on the entire population under study, but case-control studies typically include only individuals with a specific characteristic, with a sample, often a tiny minority, of the rest of the population. A cross-sectional study is one in which subjects are sampled without respect to disease status and are studied at a particular point in time, as in a random-sample health survey. |
| Case series | A report about a small group of similar cases. Typically, they are the clinical route to definition and recognition of disease entities and to the formulation of hypotheses. |
| **Experimental** | |
| Randomized controlled trials (RCTs) | RCTs are studies that measure an intervention's effect by randomly assigning individuals (or groups of individuals) to an intervention group or a control group. This is the strongest study to determine a cause–effect relation that would potentially exist between treatment and outcome. |
| **Secondary Research** | |
| Meta-analysis | A subset of systematic reviews; a method for systematically combining pertinent qualitative and quantitative study data from several selected studies to develop a single conclusion that has greater statistical power. This conclusion is statistically stronger than the analysis of any single study because of increased numbers of subjects, greater diversity among subjects, or accumulated effects and results. |

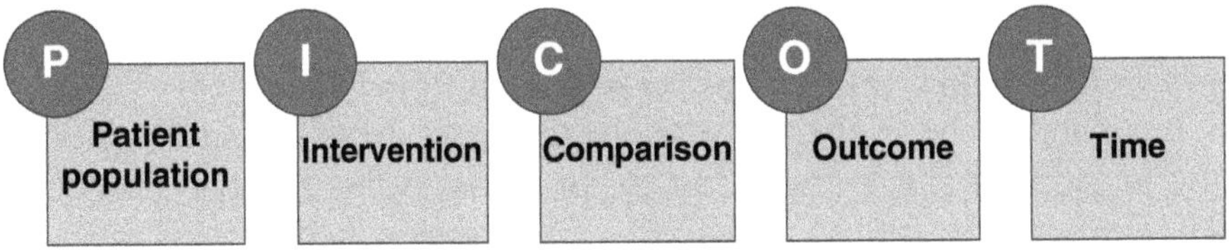

**FIGURE 3.2** PICOT. The PICOT approach is a quick and easy way to approach any research question or medical article. The method was first described by Sackett et al.[7]

The take-home message is that if PICO(T) is applicable, it is an analytic study.

### Review of the Medical Literature

As part of the introduction, it is important to review the current medical literature regarding that particular topic. This is important because it sets the stage for the relevance and applicability of that study and, more importantly, it alludes to the reason why that study was chosen. It is important to first understand the available current knowledge, cross-reference it with the current gaps in knowledge or research, and tie it into the current study and what it adds to the body of literature.

### Methods

The most important part of the Methods section is discussing the inclusion and exclusion criteria that the authors used in their study. This, coupled with the actual methodology of the study, can determine how valid and reliable results are. For results to be accurate and sound, they should arise from a nonbiased, representative sample that would in turn validate the positive or negative results of a study. In this section, one can mention the study design and how it was implemented (see Table 3.1).

### Discussion

The discussion part of the journal club presentation can be divided into two parts: discussing the results of the study and assessing the statistical methods. With respect to the statistical methods, it is important to focus on one main statistical method that the authors used and use it to convey whether they met their objectives and aims.

When presenting the results of a study, it is impossible to present every table, chart, and figure. Two to three figures should be chosen to represent the majority of the results and must be explained thoroughly with attention to the clinically significant results. Remember, a negative study is not a bad study. If a study fails to detect a relationship or elucidate a specific paradigm, then that does not mean that the study is futile. Rather, it presents further knowledge on the topic and rules out certain factors that may not be associated with it.

In assessing the statistical methods, several questions must be taken into account. It is important to first look at sample or population chosen. Does it represent an unbiased sample from which conclusions can be accurately and reliably be drawn? Is the sample or population comparable at baseline? Is the size of the sample large enough to represent enough cases that could provide conclusive inferences about a specific disease? In assessing sample size, one should also look to the power of the study. The power of a study is defined as the probability that a clinical trial will have a significant (positive) result—that is, that it will have a $P$ value of less than the specified significance level (usually 5%). In other words, it is the probability that the test will reject the null hypothesis when the null hypothesis is false (i.e., the probability of not committing a type II error, or making a false negative decision). In layman's terms, is the probability of the test reporting a statistically significant effect for a real effect of a given magnitude? If an effect has a certain size, how likely are we to discover it? Sample size and $P$ value both affect the power of the study and in turn aid in determining whether the study is statistically significant.

## Conclusion

This part of the journal club presentation is the most important with respect to individual contribution. It allows the presenter to share his or her interpretation and questions regarding the study. This is where the club assesses the relevance of the article as to whether it is *clinically* significant even though it may be statistically significant. It allows participants to analyze whether it is a feasible study and if it can be applied in clinical practice. If so, what would the economic burden associated with it be? There may be numerous studies that show that a particular diagnostic modality is highly sensitive and specific in detecting a disease, but they may be too expensive and cumbersome to be applied as a screening tool. The relevance and statistical significance of the study can also be measured by the grade and level of evidence that the study represents (Table 3.2 and Table 3.3). RCTs are typically the highest level of evidence, and data derived from them tend to represent grade A recommendations given that they are the most unbiased, controlled, blinded studies that typically confer a large sample size and contain data over a long period of time (Fig. 3.3).

The internal validity of the study should also be assessed. Did the authors rule out chance, bias, and confounding factors? Was there an external funding source? If so, what was its contribution? Not every therapeutic trial that is funded by a pharmaceutical company is deemed

**TABLE 3.2** Levels of Evidence.

| Level | Description | Examples |
|---|---|---|
| I | Evidence from at least one randomized controlled trial (RCT) or meta-analysis of RCTs | |
| II | Nonrandomized controlled trial | Prospective (cohort or outcomes) study with an internal control group or a systematic review of prospective, controlled trials |
| III | Observational studies with controls | Retrospective, time series, case control |
| IV | Observational studies without controls | Cohorts, case series without controls |
| V | Expert opinion | |

"bias." It is important to assess the funding source's contribution. If it merely supplied the finance but a separate group of investigators conducted and analyzed the study, then the results of the study can represent valid data. The external validity of the study can also be assessed by asking whether the study is feasible: Would the results change your practice? How does this fit into what we already know about the subject?

You can also comment about the importance of the article and why it was chosen. This can be commented on in the introduction as well as in the conclusion. Was it an emerging topic, pioneer procedure, or recent advancement? Did it include controversy about different regimens or inconclusive data? How does this fit our current knowledge? (refer to current practice, previous beliefs, or previous studies).

**TABLE 3.3** Grading Recommendations.

| Grade | Description |
|---|---|
| A | Directly based on category I evidence |
| B | Directly based on category II/III evidence or extrapolated recommendation from category I evidence |
| C | Directly based on category IV evidence or extrapolated recommendation from category II/III evidence |
| D | Directly based on category V evidence or inconsistent or inconclusive studies of any level |

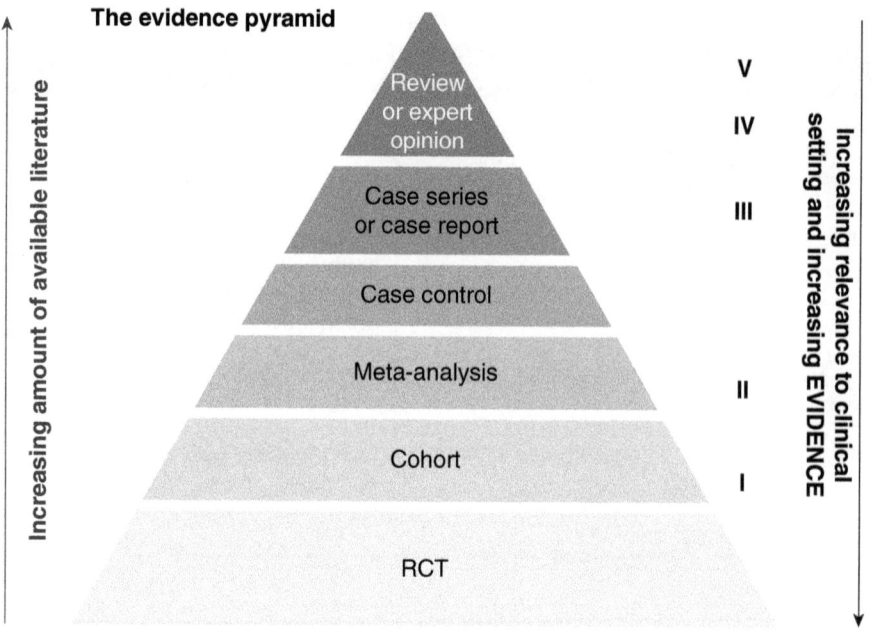

**FIGURE 3.3** The evidence pyramid. Randomized controlled trials (RCTs) represent the highest level of evidence and clinical relevance on the evidence pyramid but represent a minute amount of the available literature.

A good strategy to adopt when analyzing a study is to come up with three strengths and three weaknesses of the study. The strengths of the study can be apparent by referring to the overall effect and statistical or clinical significance. When assessing the weaknesses of a study, one can refer to specific weaknesses inherent to the study design (Table 3.4) or to author-specific weakness that may lie within the funding source, population sampling, biases, nonblinding, nonrandomization, and so on.

Finally, to conclude the presentation, the journal club should discuss either certain questions about the study such as whether the authors could have used different methodological designs or different population samples that would have brought on more solid statistically and clinically significant results. Additionally, the club may end with points for future research that were not addressed in the study.

## HOW TO CRITICALLY APPRAISE AN ARTICLE

Critical appraisal is a systematic process used to identify the strengths and weaknesses of a research article in order to assess the usefulness and validity of research findings. Numerous critical appraisal tools can

**TABLE 3.4** Potential Biases and Limitations Based on Study Design.

| Study Design | Biases and Limitations |
|---|---|
| Cross-sectional | No way to establish temporal relationship exposure and outcome measured at the same time<br>Selection bias<br>Self-reporting bias<br>Response bias |
| Case control | Selection bias (of cases and controls)<br>Recall bias<br>Questionable temporal relationship (decrease exposure before outcome) |
| Cohort | Selection bias<br>Loss to follow-up<br>Change in habits over time |
| Experimental design | Selection bias<br>Loss to follow-up<br>Improper or biased randomization procedures<br>Inadequate blinding of participants and investigators to exposure or treatment |

be used, some which are specific to the type of study under question. The most important components of a critical appraisal are an evaluation of the appropriateness of the study design for the research question and a careful assessment of the key methodological features of this design. The following questions were taken from an article by Young et al.[5] on how to appraise an article and are useful to keep in mind when reading a scientific article.

## Ten Questions to Ask When Critically Appraising a Research Article

1. Is the study question relevant?

2. Does the study add anything new?

3. What type of research question is being asked?

4. Was the study design appropriate for the research question?

5. Did the study methods address the most important potential sources of bias?

6. Was the study performed according to the original protocol?

7. Does the study test a stated hypothesis?

8. Were the statistical analyses performed correctly?

9. Do the data justify the conclusions?

10. Are there any conflicts of interest?

The following lists serve as checklists for critically appraising an article based on the specific type of article.

## Systemic Reviews and Meta-Analyses

1. Were all relevant studies included (i.e., was the search comprehensive, did it exclude articles on the basis of publication status or language, and was the potential for publication bias assessed)?

2. Were selected articles appraised and data extracted by two independent reviewers?

3. Was sufficient detail provided about the primary studies, including descriptions of the patients, interventions, and outcomes?

4. Was the quality of the primary studies assessed?

5. Did the researchers assess the appropriateness of combining results to calculate a summary measure?

## Randomized Controlled Trials

1. Was the process of treatment allocation truly random?

2. Would participants have been able to know or guess their treatment allocation?

3. Were participants and researchers "blinded" to participants' treatment group?

4. Were outcomes assessed objectively?

5. Were all participants who were randomly allocated a treatment accounted for in the final analysis?

6. Were all participants' data analyzed in the group to which they were randomly allocated?

## Cohort Study

1. Is the study prospective or retrospective?

2. Is the cohort representative of a defined group or population?

# JOURNAL CLUB WORKSHEET

Article Identifiers (Title, Author, Journal, Year):

_____

_____


## INTRODUCTION

1. **Study Type**
   a. Meta-analysis ❏
   b. Cross-sectional ❏
   c. Controlled trial ❏
      i. Randomized ❏
      ii. Nonrandomized ❏
   d. Cohort ❏
      i. Prospective ❏     Retrospective ❏
   e. Editorials, letters, opinions ❏
   f. Systematic reviews ❏
   g. Case control ❏
   h. Case series ❏
      i. Animal research ❏

2. **Type of question/problem: Circle one**
   Therapy    Prevention    Diagnosis    Etiology    Prognosis

3. **Define your question according to PICO:**
   a. Patient or problem: _____
   b. Intervention: _____
   c. Comparison: _____
   d. Outcome: _____

4. **Methods:**
   a. Double blind ❏
   b. Open label ❏
   c. Double dummy ❏
   d. Single blind ❏
   e. Other: ❏ _____

*(Continued)*

(*Continued*)

| Inclusion Criteria | Exclusion Criteria |
|---|---|
| _____ | _____ |
| _____ | _____ |
| _____ | _____ |
| _____ | _____ |
| _____ | _____ |
| _____ | _____ |

**Description**

_____

_____

_____

_____

_____

_____

## DISCUSSION

5. **Results**

_____

_____

_____

_____

6. **Statistics**

   a. Is the sample size adequate enough?          Yes ❑     No ❑

   _____

   _____

   b. Is the power adequate to answer the study question? Yes ❑ No ❑

   _____

   _____

   c. Are the study groups' characteristics comparable at baseline?

   Yes ❑     No ❑

   _____

   _____

   d. Was the population sample they chose appropriate to the question asked?          Yes ❑     No ❑

   _____

   _____

e. What is the main statistical method they used, and what did it show?

_____

_____

## CONCLUSION

7. **Relevance**

a. What is the grade or level of evidence?

_____

_____

_____

b. Clinically applicable or significant?       Yes ❑  No ❑

_____

_____

_____

c. Cost-effective?       Yes ❑  No ❑

_____

_____

_____

d. Internal validity: Did the authors rule out **chance, bias,** and **confounding** as explanations for their findings?    Yes ❑  No ❑

_____

_____

_____

e. External validity: Is this feasible? (Would these results change your practice? How do these results fit into what we already know about this subject?):    Yes ❑  No ❑

_____

_____

_____

f. Why is this article important? Why was it chosen (e.g., emerging topic, pioneer procedure, recent advancement, controversy about different regimens, inconclusive data)? How does this fit our current knowledge? (Refer to current practice, previous beliefs, or previous studies.):

_____

_____

_____

*(Continued)*

(*Continued*)

   g. Was this study funded by an external source? If so, what was the funding source's contribution?:

_____

_____

_____

8. **Strengths of Study**　　　　　　**Weaknesses and Limitations (refer to Table 3.4)**

| Strengths of Study | Weaknesses and Limitations |
|---|---|
| _____ | _____ |
| _____ | _____ |
| _____ | _____ |
| _____ | _____ |
| _____ | _____ |

9. Points to be raised during discussion (points for future research):

_____

_____

_____

_____

10. Notes

_____

_____

_____

_____

3. Were all important confounding factors identified?

4. Were all important exposures or treatments, potential confounding factors, and outcomes measured accurately and objectively in all members of the cohort?

5. Were there important losses to follow-up?

6. Were participants followed up for a sufficient length of time?

## Case-Control Study

1. Were the cases clearly defined?

2. Were the cases representative of a defined population?

3. How were the controls selected, and were they drawn from the same population as the cases?

4. Were study measures identical for cases and controls?

5. Were study measures objective or subjective, and is recall bias likely if they were subjective?

## Cross-Sectional Study

1. Was the study sample clearly defined?

2. Was a representative sample achieved (e.g., was the response rate sufficiently high)?

3. Were all relevant exposures, potential confounding factors, and outcomes measured accurately?

4. Were patients with a wide range of severity of disease assessed?

## Case Study

1. Were cases identified prospectively or retrospectively?

2. Are the cases a representative sample (e.g., a consecutive series of individuals recruited from multiple centers) and similar to patients in your practice?

3. Were all relevant exposures, potential confounding factors, and outcomes measured accurately?

The journal club worksheet serves as an initial reference that may guide you in your initial approach to understanding an article.

References

1. Ely JW, Osheroff JA, Chambliss ML, Ebell MH, Rosenbaum ME. Answering physicians' clinical questions: obstacles and potential solutions. *J Am Med Inform Assoc.* 2005;12(2):217-224.

2. Gorman PN, Helfand M. Information seeking in primary care: how physicians choose which clinical questions to pursue and which to leave unanswered. *Med Decis Making.* 1995;15(2):113.

3. Chambliss ML, Conley J. Answering clinical questions. *J Fam Pract.* 1996;43(2): 140-144.

4. Currie LM, Graham M, Allen M, Bakken S, Patel V, Cimino JJ. Clinical information needs in context: an observational study of clinicians while using a clinical information system. *AMIA Annu Symp Proc.* 2003:190-194.

5. Young JM, Solomon MJ. How to critically appraise an article. *Nat Clin Pract Gastroenterol Hepatol.* 2009;6(2):81-92.

6. Wilton NK, Slim AM. Application of the principles of evidence-based medicine to patient care. *South Med J.* 2012;105(3):136-143.

7. Sackett DL, Richardson WS, Rosenberg W, Haynes RB. *Evidence-Based Medicine: How to Practice and Teach EBM.* New York: Churchill Livingston; 1997.

8. Flemming K. Critical appraisal. 2. Searchable questions. *NT Learn Curve.* 1999; 3(2):6-7.

9. Armstrong EC. The well-built clinical question: the key to finding the best evidence efficiently. *World Med J.* 1999;98(2):25-28.

10. Timm DF, Banks DE, McLarty J. Critical appraisal process: step-by-step. *South Med J.* 2012;105(3):144-148.

11. Huang X, Lin J, Demner-Fushman D. Evaluation of PICO as a knowledge representation for clinical questions. *AMIA Annu Symp Proc.* 2006;2006:359-363.

12. Stone PW. Popping the (PICO) question in research and evidence-based practice. *Appl Nurs Res.* 2002;15(3):197-198.

# 4

# HOW TO INTERPRET RESEARCH

## *Easy statistics*

*With contributions from Fahed Barakat, BSc, MBBS*

Statistics is probably the most feared topic in the realm of medicine among medical students and residents. It encompasses a rarely charted field that ironically is the basis for the majority of our clinical decision making. To use evidence-based medicine (EBM) in daily practice, it is important to understand whether recent clinical studies are significant enough to be implemented in our daily lives. This chapter provides the statistical knowledge needed in order to understand what statistical tests are used and how to interpret the final results.

## BASIC STATISTICS

When gathering data for a certain study, it is entered individually into a database, one observation at a time. The material is recorded as a set of variables. Statistics involves comparing information within these variables to answer the research question.

### Type of Data
- Continuous (measured): Continuous data take any value within a range such as height, weight, or age.
- Discrete (categorical): Data belong to a restricted number of classes.
  - Binary: There are only two possible options (e.g., dead or alive, yes or no).
  - Nominal: There is no particular order in categories (e.g., ethnicity, occupation).
  - Ordinal: Categories can be ordered (e.g., age group, smoking status: non, ex, current).

## Center of Data

When summarizing numerical observed data from a study sample, it is useful to obtain a value for the center of the data. This can take several forms:[1,2]

- **Mean:** Also known as the average and more accurately known as the arithmetic mean. This is the most commonly used statistic, but its use may not always be appropriate.
- **Median:** The halfway point of the variable. The numbers are all rearranged in ascending or descending order, and the value that lies in the middle is the median (when there is an odd number of observations). If two values lie in the middle (when number of observations is even), the average of the two is considered the median.
- **Mode:** This is the most frequently observed number (not used often; more relevant in discrete data).

The mean is much more sensitive to outliers (an observation that is numerically distant to the rest of the data) the median. Hence, the choice of which measure to use as the center of data depends on the spread and distribution of the variable (Table 4.1).

## Spread of Data

While assessing data, how wide do the rest of the observations spread or disperse around the calculated center (mean, median, mode)? This is a measure of precision.

- **Range:** This is the difference between the maximum and minimum values.
- **Interquartile range (IQR):** This is numerical range of a variable that contains the middle 50% of the sample. The upper limit of

**TABLE 4.1** Describing Data.*

| | Outlier Not Included | Outlier Included |
|---|---|---|
| Mean | $(1+4+4+10+3+6+9+4+4+2+2+7+4+6+8)/15 = 4.93$ | $(1+4+4+10+3+6+9+4+4+2+2+7+4+6+8+30)/16 = 6.5$ |
| Median | *1, 2, 2, 3, 4, 4, 4, 4, 4, 6, 6, 7, 8, 9, 10* <br> The midway observation is 4. | *1, 2, 2, 3, 4, 4, 4, 4, 6, 6, 7, 8, 9, 10, 30* <br> The average of the middle 2 observations is 4. |
| Mode | 4 is the most frequently occurring observation. | 4 remains the most frequently occurring observation. |

*This table summarizes statistics derived from the following sample: {1, 4, 4, 10, 3, 6, 9 4, 4, 2, 2, 7, 4, 6, 8}. 30 is used as an outlying observation.

**TABLE 4.2** Range, Interquartile Range, Standard
Deviation, and Variance.*

|  | Outlier Not Included | Outlier Included |
|---|---|---|
| Range | Minimum = 1<br>Maximum = 10<br>Range = 1–10 | Minimum = 1<br>Maximum = 30<br>Range = 1–30 |
| Interquartile range | 1, 2, 2, 3, 4, 4, 4, 4, 4, 6, 6, 7,<br>8, 9, 10<br>Lower quartile = 3<br>Upper quartile = 7<br>Interquartile range = 7 – 3 = 4 | 1, 2, 2, 3, 4, 4, 4, 4, 4, 6, 6, 7, 8,<br>9, 10, 30<br>Lower quartile = 3.5<br>Upper quartile = 7.5<br>Interquartile range = 7.5 – 3.5 = 4 |
| Standard deviation | 2.66 | 6.77 |
| Variance | 7.07 | 45.87 |

*This table summarizes statistics derived from the following sample: {1, 4, 4, 10, 3, 6, 9 4, 4, 2, 2, 7, 4, 6, 8}. 30 is used as an outlying observation.

the range is the upper quartile (75th percentile), and the lower limit is the lower quartile (25th percentile).

- Standard deviation (SD): The above measures of dispersion only consider the rank of the values of the observations. SD also takes the magnitude of the observation into account. We consider the distance each observation is from the calculated *mean* value of the data.
- Variance: This is the square of the SD.

The SD and variance are sensitive to outliers, but the IQR is not (Table 4.2).

## Presenting Basic Data

Discrete data can be easily interpreted from a contingency table or a bar diagram. Here we will focus on presenting continuous data graphically.[3]

- Histogram: These are similar to bar charts. Bars are constructed for intervals of data, and the area rather than the height represents the frequency of observations within that interval.
- Box and whisker plot: Also called a box plot. It consists of a rectangular box oriented vertically (sometimes horizontally) representing the distribution of the middle 50% of the data (IQR) with a horizontal line within it identifying the median. The whiskers that extend upward and downward display the variability

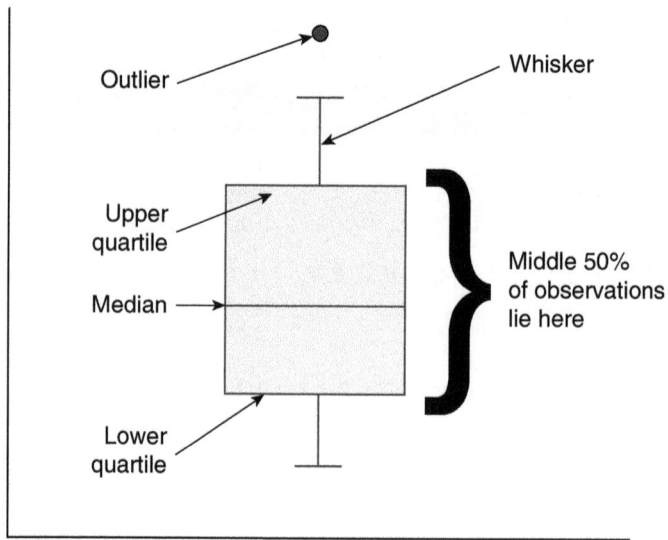

**FIGURE 4.1** Box and whisker plot.

in the data outside the realm of the middle quartiles. However, different box plot uses different reference points for their hinges (i.e., whisker limits). Outliers are sometimes plotted as individual points (Fig. 4.1).

### Distribution of Data

- Symmetric: A symmetric distribution is one in which the right and left halves are mirror images of each other (possess the same shape). If the distribution of data is symmetric, then the mean and the median are the same value.
- Skewed: If asymmetric, it is described as skewed. Whereas right skewness means that the tail is elongated on the right side, left skewness is left rail elongation. In this distribution, the mean is located away from the median in the direction of skewness.

In the initial phase of statistical analysis, one purely describes the data obtained, and this is summarized in a table (baseline characteristics). Discrete data are presented simply as frequencies and percentages. However, when displaying continuous data in a table, which measurement of center and spread of data should be used (mean and median or SD and IQR)? Each continuous variable is analyzed separately. If the variable proves to have an approximately symmetrical distribution, the mean and SD are used. If the variable's distribution is obviously skewed, the median and IQR may be more valuable.

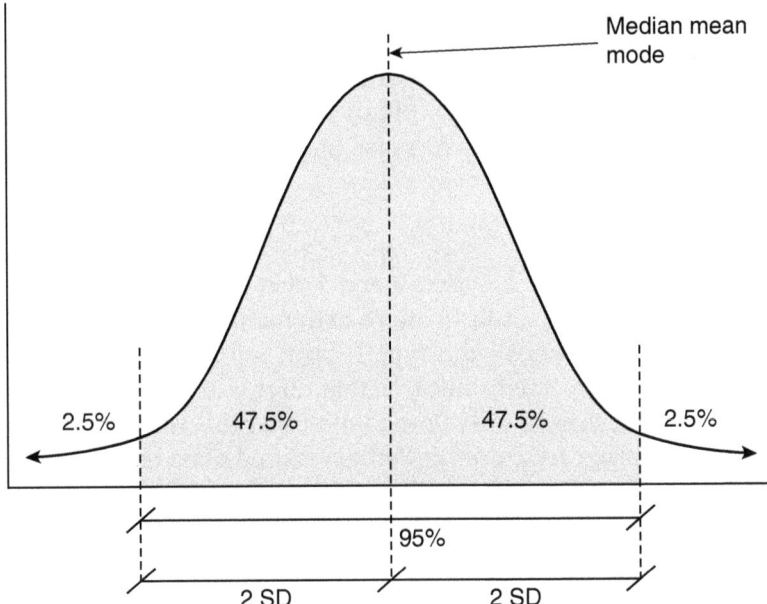

**FIGURE 4.2** Normal distribution curve.

## Normal Distribution

A normal (Gaussian) distribution is a symmetrical, bell-shaped distribution in which the median, mode, and mean coincide, and is absolutely
continuous (no maximum and minimum values). It is extremely important in statistics, mainly because of the central limit theorem (CLT).
The CLT states that no matter what the original distribution shape of a
sample, as the number of observations increases, the distribution tends
to a normal distribution. Roughly 95% of observations lie within 2 SDs
on either side of the mean (Fig. 4.2).

## ASSESSING SIGNIFICANCE

The reason we carry out medical research is to extrapolate our findings
to the general population. A sample is obtained from the population.
A statistic is calculated from the collected data. Does this mean that this
corresponds to the mean of the population? The answer is no. We must
know the precision of the estimate and how likely it is that we obtained
the value because of chance.

### Null Hypothesis

The null hypothesis is the hypothesis that there is no difference between
two groups or there is no treatment effect. During statistical analysis,

a statistically significant test rejects the null hypothesis and therefore accepts the alternative hypothesis (difference between groups or a treatment effect). However, using standard (or frequentist) statistical theory, we can never accept the null hypothesis even though the observed value was statistically insignificant. Absence of evidence is not equivalent to the evidence of absence.

## P Value

The P value is a number between 0 and 1 that represents the chance of obtaining the observed result or more extreme in magnitude if the null hypothesis is true (also called a type I error; see section on Power). In other words, if we observe from a trial that there is a treatment effect with a P value of 0.03; there is a 3% probability that this value was obtained by chance. The arbitrary cutoff of $P < 0.05$ is used quite regularly to identify a statistically significant result. Authors note the chosen cutoff of statistical significance in the statistical methods section of the article.[1,2]

## Confidence Intervals

As mentioned earlier, we cannot use one observed value to extrapolate to the general population. A range of possible true population values should be presented based on the information obtained from the observed sample. Generally, a 95% confidence interval (CI) is constructed surrounded the observed result. Statistically speaking, the following explanation of this interval is not correct; however, it is simpler to understand the concept with it. A 95% CI makes you 95% confident that the true population value lies within the limits of the constructed interval. If the null value (0 if difference, 1 if ratio) lies within the constraints of this interval, we cannot reject the null hypothesis. However, if the null value lies outside the interval, then $P < 0.05$, and the null hypothesis is rejected. As expected, a narrow CI is preferred, suggesting a precise estimate of the population value.

## Power

There are two types of errors that can occur when interpreting results of a study:

- Type I error: Denoted as $\alpha$. This is the probability of obtaining a statistically significant observed result when in reality the null hypothesis is true.
- Type II error: Denoted by $\beta$. This is the probability of obtaining no significant observed result when in reality the alternative hypothesis is true.
- Power: Equivalent to 1 minus type II error (or 1-$\beta$). This is the probability of obtaining a statistically significant observed value

when in reality the alternative hypothesis is true. Traditionally, researchers consider a study power of 80% to be the minimum value to detect an effect.

## ASSUMPTIONS

Data need to fit certain assumptions for certain tests to be performed. Standard tests require more assumptions to hold for a result to be interpreted correctly; otherwise, the use of that test is not valid. If certain assumptions do not fit, there are some *tricks* to make the statistical model assumptions fit. If these assumptions cannot be met, more *robust* methods are used. The literal meaning of *robust* does not hold in the statistics context. It is used to describe a statistical procedure, the validity of which is less reliant on assumptions than other standard, more frequently used alternatives. Some common assumptions are listed below.

### Independence

Observations are considered independent if the outcome of one observation is not directly or indirectly affected by another. For example, in a study comparing height in infants with daily caloric intake, the observations are considered independent if observations are not siblings, are not cared for by the same adult, and so on.

### Linearity

The variables included in the statistical model are linearly (straight line) related to each other. Using the same example as above, if the increase in caloric intake is associated with a uniform increase in infant height; the linearity assumption holds.

### Normal Distribution

This is usually an assumption for the outcome variable. The best possible way to try to adjust the variable distribution to mimic a normal distribution is by using the CLT and increasing the size of the sample. Most of the time this is not possible, so we can transform the variable to create a distribution closer to the model. The most commonly used transformation is to use the log (base e) of outcome values.

## STANDARD STATISTICAL PROCEDURES

These are tests that all require certain assumptions to be met. We will not dwell on which assumptions are required for which of these tests.[4]

## *t*-Test

The two-sample *t*-test is a statistical test that is very commonly seen in the literature. It is used to compare two defined groups with regards to a continuous variable. These can be paired or unpaired. The unpaired *t*-test can be used in the example of comparing the means of systolic blood pressure in a two group differing by gender. The paired *t*-test would be one that compares the means of systolic blood pressure of the same sample before and after use of antihypertensive medications. A *P* <0.05 suggests that there is evidence of a difference between the two groups.

## Chi-Squared of Association

The chi-squared association is used as a method of testing the association of categorical variables. A *P* <0.05 indicates that there is evidence of an association between the two variables. A similar test used for smaller samples is the Fisher's exact test.

## Pearson's Correlation

A method used to test association between two continuous variables. A correlation coefficient is calculated. It takes on values between −1 and 1. If the value is positive, then as one variable increases, the other increases. If the value is negative, as one variable increases, the other decreases. A value of zero means there is no linear relation. Values of 0.5 to 0.6 imply a moderate correlation, 0.6 to 0.7 suggest a good correlation, and 0.7 to 0.8 suggest an excellent correlation. It is unusual but possible to find correlation coefficients higher than 0.8 in magnitude. A coefficient of 1 infers a perfectly straight line relation, which is never seen.

## Linear Regression

This is a statistical model that is the foundation of many more complex models, including Cox, logistic, and log linear regression. Here we will only briefly discuss linear regression. Linear regression is used when the outcome variable is continuous.

- Simple linear regression: This method constructs a best-fit line through the observed data of the outcome variable against one predictor variable or covariate (e.g., age, gender, smoking status, treatment). Simple linear regression calculates a regression coefficient, which is the slope that suggests how much the outcome variable increases for every unit increase (continuous) or change in category (discrete) in the predictor variable. If we again take systolic blood pressure as an example and assume it is linearly related to age, a positive regression coefficient (say, 2) suggests that the expected systolic blood pressure increased by 2 for every 1-year increase in age in the observed sample. If the regression coefficient was negative, then the expected blood pressure is decreased by 2 for every 1-year increase in age. A regression coefficient of 0 means that there is no association between the outcome and predictor variable. In the case of a discrete predictor variable (gender), a regression coefficient can be calculated for being male (say, 5). Therefore, we can conclude the systolic blood pressure is 5 units higher in males compared with females.

- Multiple linear regression: Also called multivariable linear regression. It is very useful at identifying possible confounding. If in our example above, we notice that the male group was on average older than the female group, we would expect that the overall effect of gender on blood pressure was overestimated. Therefore, multiple linear regression is used to calculated *adjusted* (rather than *crude* or *marginal*) coefficients. Thus, if the regression coefficient of age is 2 when both age and gender are included in the regression model, the interpretation is as follows. For every 1-year increase in age, we observed a 2-unit increase in systolic blood pressure, adjusting for gender (or keeping gender constant).

Results obtained after using the above tests would be invalid if the assumptions of the corresponding procedures are not met. More robust methods include the Mann-Whitney U-test, Spearman rank correlation, permutation procedures, bootstrapping, sandwich estimators, and so on. Unfortunately, there is a tradeoff between robustness of a test and its power.

## INTERPRETING STUDY-SPECIFIC STATISTICS

### Statistics in Cross-Sectional Studies[5]

- Prevalence: The proportion of people who have a certain exposure or outcome of interest at a certain point in time
- Prevalence ratio: Ratio of prevalence between two groups. If the HIV prevalence ratio of population A to B is 1.5, the prevalence of HIV is 50% higher in population A. If the prevalence ratio was less than 1 (say, 0.8), then the prevalence of HIV in population a is ([1 - 0.8] * 100) 20% lower than in population B. A prevalence ratio of 1 suggests there is no difference in ratio between the two populations.
- Odds ratios (ORs): See the next section.

## Statistics in Case-Control Studies

- Prevalence
- Odds of exposure: Ratio of exposed to unexposed
- OR of exposure: Ratio of odds of exposure in the diseased group (cases) to odds of exposure in the nondiseased (controls) group. Interpretation is similar to that for a prevalence ratio.

## Statistics in Cohort Studies

- Prevalence
- Cumulative Incidence (risk): The proportion of new cases that develop over a fixed period of time from a population of individuals at risk. If numbers are too small, values are presented per 1,000. Because follow-up time can vary among individuals in a study, rate can sometimes be more appropriate.
- Rate: Proportion of new cases that develop a disease out of a population of individual's time at risk
- Risk/rate ratio: Ratio of risk/rate in exposed group to that in the unexposed group. Also called *relative risk* (RR). Interpretation is similar to that of the prevalence ratio.
- Absolute risk/rate difference: The difference in risk/rate between the exposed and the unexposed groups. Whereas positive values imply an absolute increase in risk in the exposed group, negative values imply an absolute reduction in risk in the exposed group. Can also be called *attributable risk*. It is the measure of additional risk attributed by the exposure.
- Number needed to treat: The number of individuals who needed to be treated to prevent one death or event. It is the reciprocal of attributable risk (1/attributable risk).
- Odds of disease: Ratio of diseased to nondiseased
- OR of disease: Ratio of odds of disease in the exposed group to odds of disease in the unexposed group

Note that the OR of exposure and the OR of disease use the same formula; however, they are interpreted differently in case-control studies (OR of exposure) and cohort studies (OR of disease). Although risk, rate, and ORs can be used in cohort studies, risk is relatively more commonly used (Fig. 4.3).

## Statistics in Randomized Controlled Trials

- Risk, rate, and OR: Except we substitute the group names from exposed and unexposed groups to intervention and control groups.

| | Disease PRESENT | Disease ABSENT |
|---|---|---|
| Test POSITIVE | **A**<br><br>True positives | **B**<br><br>False positives |
| Test NEGATIVE | **C**<br><br>False negatives | **D**<br><br>True negatives |

| | Disease PRESENT | Disease ABSENT | Total |
|---|---|---|---|
| Exposure PRESENT | **A** | **B** | **A+B** |
| Exposure ABSENT | **C** | **D** | **C+D** |
| Total | **A+C** | **B+D** | **N** |

Sensitivity: A/(A+C)
Specificity: D/(D+B)
Pretest probability: (A+C)/(A+B+C+D)
PPV*: A/A+B
NPV**: D/C+D

**A**

Odds ratio: $\dfrac{A/C}{B/D} = \dfrac{AD}{BC}$
Relative risk: $\dfrac{A/(A+B)}{C/(C+D)}$
Attributable risk: A/(A+B)–C/(C+D)

**B**

**FIGURE 4.3** Statistical Punnett squares representing simple calculations for sensitivity, specificity, odds ratio, relative risk, attributable risk, and positive predictive value (PPV) and negative predictive value (NPV).

## GRAPHICAL PRESENTATION

In addition to understanding the terminology and the numbers, diagrams are very informative in medical articles. However, much of this information is missed if one does not know how to interpret these figures.

### Survival Curves

Survival data confer an intricate and complex analysis due to numerous factors, namely censoring (subjects lost to follow-up or not reaching the "event" by the end of the study period) and highly skewed duration distributions (some subjects have a very large duration and others have a relatively short duration).[6,7] Objectives for survival analysis curves are:

- To model the survival pattern over a period of time
- To investigate factors that influence the duration of survival
- To compare two or more modalities for survival pattern
- To estimate future survival of individuals or groups with specified features.

Numerous methods have been employed to analyze such data; one of the most common ones is the Kaplan-Meier curve.

- Kaplan-Meier curves: This method is used when subjects are continuously observed and the exact duration or time of drop out is

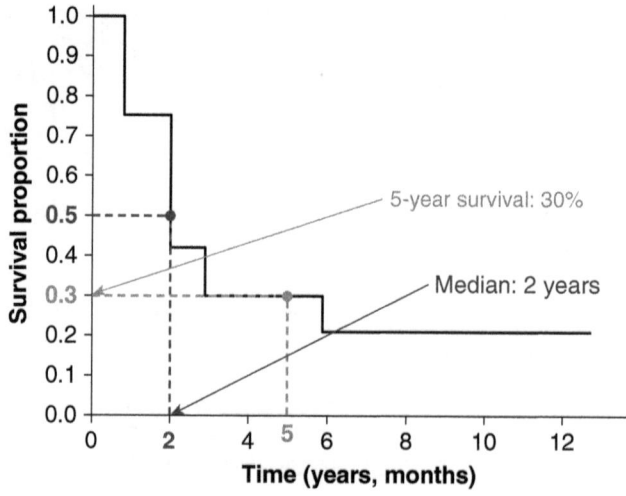

**FIGURE 4.4** Kaplan-Meier Curve basics. The Kaplan-Meier curve consists of an *x*-axis depicting time (years or months) and a *y*-axis depicting the survival proportion. The median survival is the time at which the percentage surviving is 50%. The curve steps down at each death and is flat in between deaths, which leads to the classic staircase appearance.

known. To interpret such a graph, one must understand the different elements of the graph (Fig. 4.4):

- General setup: The time that the curve covers is broken up into intervals, and then the percentage surviving at the start of any interval is equal to the probability of surviving each of the preceding intervals all multiplied together. First, suppose that after 2 years, the survival curve has reached 60%. Then suppose that during the third year, 10% *of the surviving* patients die, leaving 90% surviving. Consequently, at the start of the fourth year, you can calculate that 90% of 60% = 54% of patients are still alive.
- Staircase appearance: The general shape of this survival curve is a staircase shape that mimics the actual experience of a study population. Thus, the curve steps down at each death and is flat in between deaths, leading to the classic staircase appearance.
- Horizontal lines: Survival duration for that interval
- Vertical lines: Partly used for visual aesthetics (to make horizontal lines easier to see) but also represent the cumulative probability as the curve advances
- *y*-axis: Proportion of people surviving
- *x*-axis: The time after the start of the observation. It is important to understand that even if they started observing or treating different

patients at different times, the curve represents the experience of each patient from the time that observation or treatment started for that patient. For example, if two patients start 4 months apart in a clinical trial and each survives 1 year after they start, they are both considered as survivors at 1 year in the survival curve.

- The **median survival** is the time at which the percentage surviving is 50%.
- Censoring data: Mathematically removing a patient from the curve at the end of his or her follow-up time. The aim is to produce the most accurate possible survival curve, taking into account all information available. When a patient is censored, the curve does not take a step down as it does when a patient dies. In fact, unless the curve has tick marks to show where patients were censored, there is nothing to tell you where a patient was censored. Because censoring an observation reduces the number of patients contributing to the curve, each death after censoring represents a higher proportion of the remaining population. Hence, every downward step will be a slightly larger than it would be if individuals were not censored.

Different types of survival curves include (Fig. 4.5):
- Graphs ending in a plateau: These curves suggest that patients are being cured or no "deaths" have occurred because no downward step occurred on the graph. Two graphs may plateau at 6 years, where one demonstrates an initially steeper slope (indicating a lower probability that these patients would survive at 6 years of follow-up) versus one with a gentler slope indicating a higher probability of patients being alive at 6 years. Figure 4.5A demonstrates a flat curve that starts to plateau after 8 years/months at approximately 60% survival. This survival curve would have been more ominous if the slope was steeper and started to plateau at 10%.
- Curves that descend to zero: These curves imply that no one (or almost no one) survives the full period of follow-up. Even curves that reach zero may differ in their shape. Examining the slope is extremely important because two curves that both reach the $x$-axis can be interpreted differently based on their slope. If the slope is flatter, then even though there are ultimately no survivors, people lived quite a few years (as depicted by Fig. 4.5B).
- Comparison curves: When interpreting two survival curves for two or more different treatments, one should take into account the slope of the line and the trend (whether it plateaus or reaches zero). If one curve is continuously "above" the other, as with

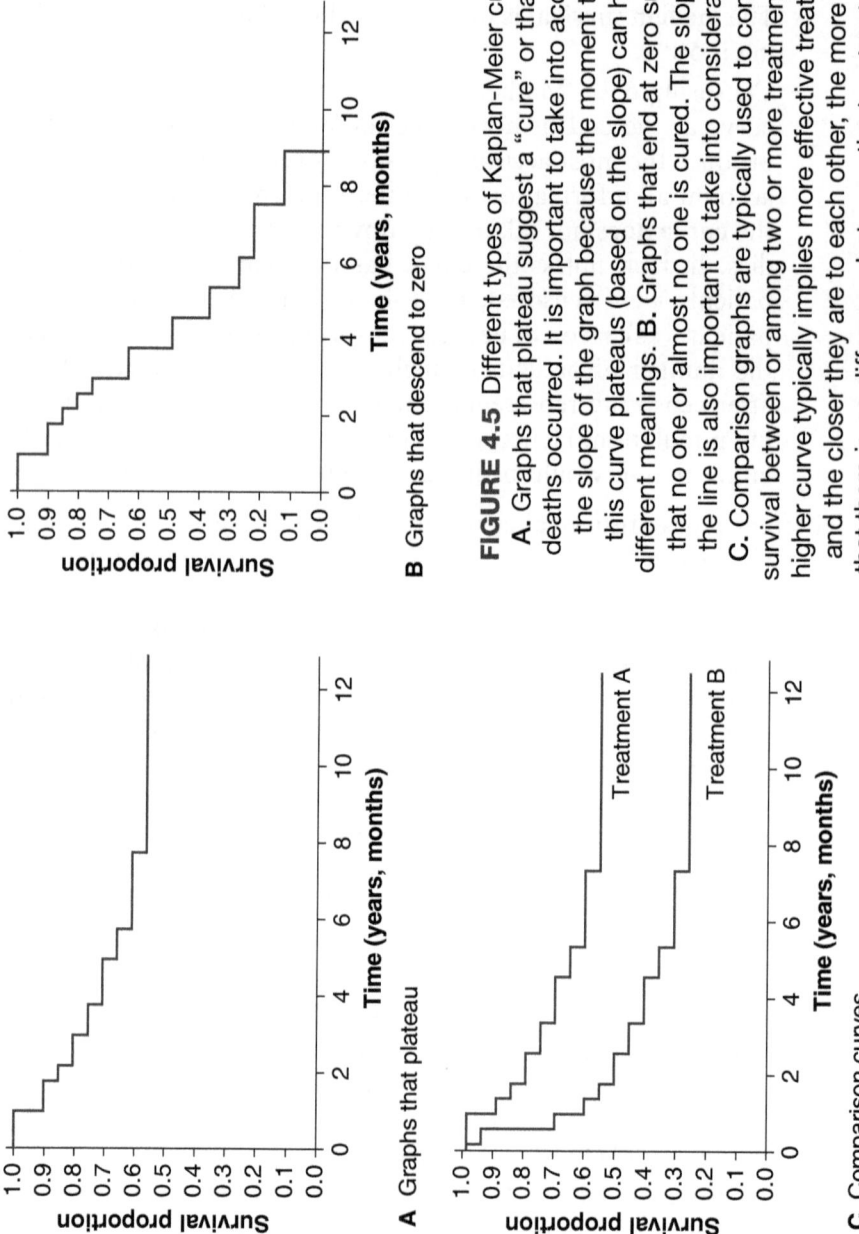

**FIGURE 4.5** Different types of Kaplan-Meier curves. **A.** Graphs that plateau suggest a "cure" or that no deaths occurred. It is important to take into account the slope of the graph because the moment that this curve plateaus (based on the slope) can have different meanings. **B.** Graphs that end at zero suggest that no one or almost no one is cured. The slope of the line is also important to take into consideration. **C.** Comparison graphs are typically used to compare survival between or among two or more treatments. The higher curve typically implies more effective treatments, and the closer they are to each other, the more likely that there is no difference between the two treatments.

the curves in Figure 4.5C, the conclusion is that the treatment associated with the higher curve was more effective for these patients. Closer curves indicate no or little difference between the treatments. Figure 4.5C shows that treatment A is superior to treatment B because approximately 60% are alive and continue to be alive at 8 years with treatment A, but only 30% remain alive and stay alive by 8 years with treatment B.

- Cox regression: Cox curves are used to delineate the role of covariates that affect the duration of survival.[3,6,7] Covariates include the treatment a patient received, the patient's age or weight, or the dosage of a drug. This curve typically uses the hazard ratio. The hazard ratio is the probability of dying (or experiencing the event in question) conditional that the patient has survived up to a given point in time. In other words, it is the instantaneous chance of death (or event); however, it does not depend on time.[7] The proportional hazards method computes a coefficient for each predictor variable that indicates the direction and degree of flexing that the predictor has on the survival curve. Zero means that a variable has no effect on the curve (it is not a predictor at all); a positive variable indicates that larger values of the variable are associated with greater mortality. Knowing these coefficients, we could construct a "customized" survival curve for any particular combination of predictor values. More important, the method provides a measure of the sampling error associated with each predictor's coefficient.[2]

## Receiver Operating Characteristics Curve

To better understand receiver operating characteristic (ROC) curves, it is crucial to be familiar with some terminology:[8]

- Sensitivity: The proportion of patients *with* disease who test positive or the proportion of correctly identified true positives
- TP/[TP + FN]*
- Specificity: The proportion of patients *without* disease who test negative. Or the proportion of correctly identified true negatives: TN/[TN + FP]
- Positive predictive value (PPV): The probability of actually having the disease with a positive test result: TP/[TP + FP]*
- Negative predictive value (NPV): The probability of actually *not* having the disease with a negative test result: TN/[TN + FN]

---

*True positives (TP), False negatives (FN), True negatives (TN), False positives (FP).

**TABLE 4.3** Usefulness and Quality of a Test.

| Sensitivity | Likelihood That the Diagnostic Test Will Indicate the Presence of Disease When the Disease is Actually Present (True Positive Rate) | Quality of a Test |
|---|---|---|
| Specificity | Likelihood that the diagnostic test will indicate the absence of disease when the disease is actually absent | Quality of a test |
| Positive predictive value (PPV) | Likelihood that a positive test result actually means that the disease is present | Usefulness of a test |
| Negative predictive value (NPV) | Likelihood that a negative test result actually means that the disease is absent | Usefulness of a test |

- Pretest probability: The estimated likelihood of disease before the test is done. If a defined population of patients is being evaluated, the pretest probability is equal to the **prevalence** of disease in the population. It is the proportion of total patients who have the disease: [TP + FN]/[TP + FP + TN + FN] (Table 4.3).

Now we return to the ROC curve. It is a graphical technique describing and comparing the **accuracy of** diagnostic tests and is obtained by plotting the sensitivity of a test on the $y$-axis against 1-specificity on the $x$-axis. The area under the ROC curve provides a measure of the overall performance of a diagnostic test. The curve may be used to select optimal cutoff values for a test result, assess the diagnostic accuracy, and compare the efficacy of different tests.

Generally, when one wishes to describe whether a disease is "present" or "absent," certain cutoff values are required to satisfy disease definitions. As mentioned earlier, the sensitivity and specificity of a test depend on the chosen cutoff level separating the normal (negative) from the abnormal (positive). The ROC curve helps define what constitutes an abnormal test. Components of an ROC curve include:

- $y$-axis: Sensitivity (the proportion of true positive results) going from 0 to 1 (0%–100%); also known as "true positive rate"
- $x$-axis: 1-specificity (the proportion of false positive results) going from 0 to 1 (0%–100%)[8]; also known as "true negative rate"
- Reference line: The diagonal line extending from the lower left-hand corner to the upper right-hand corner of the graph serves as a reference line. It represents the characteristics of a test, which are completely useless at differentiating between those with

disease and those without disease.[8] Points along this line indicate that the test detects an equal number of true and false positives; that is, it does not discriminate between those with disease and those without disease.[9]

■ A **perfect test** would ideally carry a 100% specificity and a 100% sensitivity, implying that it is able to discriminate between diseased and nondiseased subjects. The closest curve that would emulate this would be one that is closer to the left hand corner.

■ Area under the curve (AUC): The AUC serves as a single measure, independent of prevalence, that summarizes the discriminative ability of a test across the full range of cutoffs. It reflects of how good the test is at distinguishing between patients with disease and those without disease. The greater the AUC, the better the test.[10] In general, the closer the AUC is to 1, the better the overall diagnostic performance of the test, and the closer it is to 0.5, the poorer the test (Fig. 4.6).

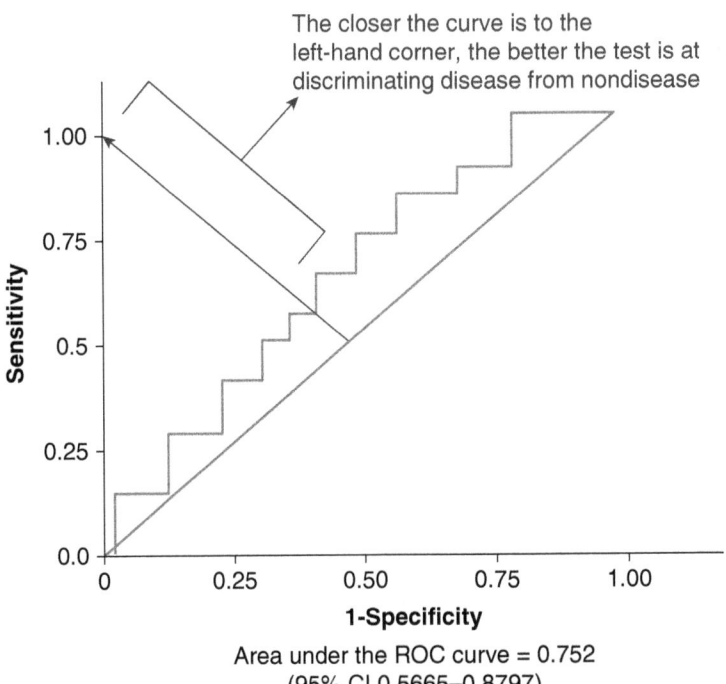

Area under the ROC curve = 0.752
(95% CI 0.5665–0.8797)

**FIGURE 4.6** The ROC (receiver operating characteristic) curve, a graphical technique for describing and comparing the accuracy of diagnostic tests, is obtained by plotting the sensitivity of a test on the *y*-axis against 1-specificity on the *x*-axis.

## Forest Plots

Many of the clinical decisions today are based on EBM derived from research studies. To maintain current medical knowledge, one would have to read an insurmountable number of medical articles published in millions of references and thousands of journals on a daily basis. To address this challenge, the systematic review method was created.[9] One of the most valuable medical articles is a metaanalysis, which is a systematic method of evaluating statistical data based on results of several independent studies of the same problem. One of the methods in analyzing such a clinical design is a forest plot.

Metaanalysis graphs are commonly displayed graphically as forest plots. The majority of metaanalyses combine data from multiple interventional studies. Some metaanalyses contain binary variables (e.g., disease vs. no disease) expressed as ratios, and others contain continuous data (e.g., serum creatinine levels) that are expressed as the "weighted mean difference" (WMD) (Fig. 4.7).

A forest plot is typically expressed in six columns with individual study data contained in rows.

1. Details of review: A small summary of the purpose or aim of the studies included with specification of the comparison and outcome measures.

2. First column: Lists the study IDs used in the meta-analysis.

3. Second and third columns: Contain the study population groups.

   a. In continuous outcome measures: The total number of participants in the group is included as N along with the mean and SD.

   b. In binary outcome measures: n is the number of participants with the outcome, and N is the total number of participants in the group.

4. Fourth column: Graphically displays the study results. The line in the middle is referred to as "the line of no effect" that illustrates no difference between the intervention/control group. This pertains to a WMD of 0 in continuous outcome measures or a RR or OR of 1 in binary outcome measures.

   a. Value axis: At the bottom of the graph; favors the intervention group based on the outcome being studied (Table 4.4).

   b. Size of boxes: Directly related to the "weighting" of the study in the meta-analysis.

5. Whiskers: Depict the CI, where the longer the whiskers, the wider the CI, and hence the less precise the study results. Cases in which there are arrows in the whiskers, illustrate that the CI is wider than there is space in the graph.

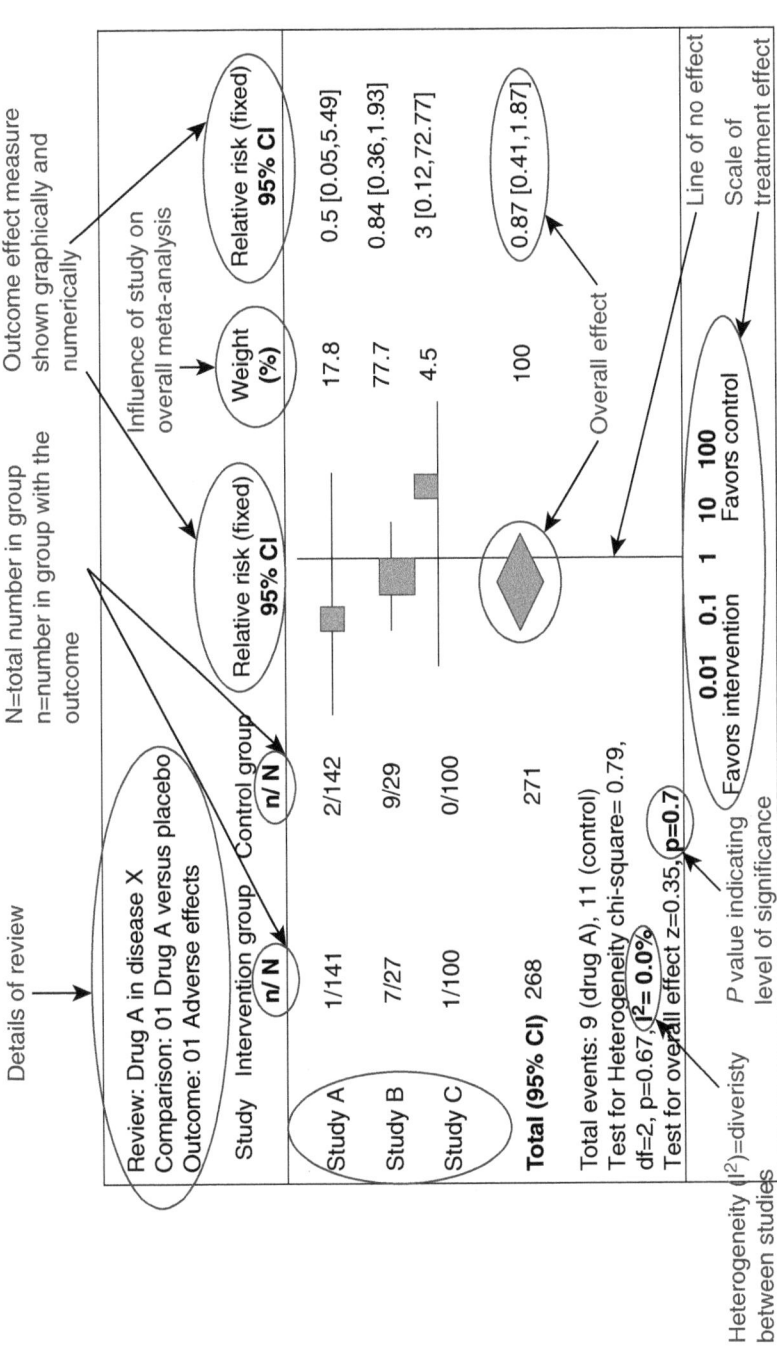

**FIGURE 4.7** The forest plot for a binary outcome measure. Metaanalysis graphs are commonly displayed graphically as forest plots. (Adapted from Ried K. Interpreting and understanding meta-analysis graphs—a practical guide. *Aust Fam Physician.* 2006;35(8):635-638.)

**TABLE 4.4** Comparison of Outcome Effects for Binary and Continuous Variables on a Forest Plot.

| Outcome Effect Measure | Binary | Continuous |
|---|---|---|
| Line of no effect | Ratios: RR or OR = 1 | Difference between means, WMD = 0 |
| If outcome is **undesirable**: heart attack | Favors intervention on **left**-hand side of scale (**ratio <1**) | Favors intervention on **left**-hand side of scale (**WMD <0**) |
| If **decreased** outcome effect measure is **desirable**: decreased blood pressure | Favors intervention on **left**-hand side of scale (**ratio <1**) | Favors intervention on **left**-hand side of scale (**WMD <0**) |
| If outcome effect measure is **desirable**: stopping smoking | Favors intervention on **right**-hand side of scale (**ratio >1**) | Favors intervention on **right**-hand side of scale (**WMD >0**) |

OR, odds ratio; RR, relative risk; WMD, weighted mean difference.

6. Weight (%): The "weighting" of an article illustrates the influence of the study on the overall results of the metaanalysis of all included studies. The higher the percentage, the bigger the box and the more influence the study has on the overall results. This is determined by the study's sample size and precision of results provided as evidenced by tighter CIs.

7. Numerical results: Either depicted as relative risk (RR) for binary outcome measures or the WMD for continuous outcome measures. They represent the numerical value of the graphically displayed result in the prior column.

8. Total study effect: This is depicted both numerically and graphically, typically in the last row. The large diamond is the graphical display of the total effect or result of the metaanalysis as a whole. The middle of the diamond corresponds to the overall effect estimate (either RR or WMD), and the width corresponds to the CI.

   a. Statistically significant metaanalysis:
      i. If the diamond does not cross 0 (WMD for continuous) or 1 (RR for binary)
      ii. $P$ value <0.05

9. Heterogeneity test ($I^2$): This value ranges between 0% and 100% and illustrates the diversity or variability between the studies. It gives an indication of how comparable the different studies are. The lower

the number, the more comparable the studies are, making the meta-analysis stronger. Another way to assess variability is to see whether the whiskers (CI) of the studies overlap; if so, it would make them more homogenous.

- Hazard ratios: Hazard ratios describe the outcome of clinical therapeutic trials to determine what extent the treatment can shorten the duration of an illness. It is the relative risk of a complication based on comparison of event rates. It can be applied to any situation in which the subjects will have different times to an event or outcome of interest. In a clinical trial in which disease resolution is the end point, the hazard ratio indicates the relative likelihood of disease resolution in treated versus control subjects at any given point in time.[10]
  - The slope of the survival curve is a measure of how rapidly subjects are dying.
  - Expression of the hazard or chance of events occurring in the treatment arm as a ratio of the hazard of the events occurring in the control arm. The term *hazard ratio* is often used interchangeably with the term *relative risk ratio* to describe results in clinical trials.
  - Calculated using a statistical technique known as survival analysis. Survival analysis keeps track of how many subjects have *not* experienced the event at a given time or during a given time interval. The data are then plotted over the entire time of the study, and the results are graphed as a decreasing curve. The curve decreases as time increases as well as the number of patients experiencing the event.
  - Roughly defined, it is "conditional instantaneous event rate calculated as a function of time."
  - A hazard ratio = 1: There is no difference in hazard between the two groups.
  - A hazard ratio greater than 1: The desired event is happening faster for the treatment group than for the control group.
  - A hazard ratio less than 1: The event of interest is happening slower for the treatment group than for the control group.
  - In general, treatment efficacy is denoted by a hazard ratio of less than 1.0 in prevention trials and a hazard ratio of greater than 1.0 in treatment trials.
  - A hazard ratio of 2 implies that at any time, twice as many patients in the active group are having an event proportionately compared with the control group. A hazard ratio of 0.5 means

**TABLE 4.5** Statistical Tests Primer.

| Statistical Test | Value | Notes |
|---|---|---|
| Confidence interval (CI) | 1. Statistically significant: if CI does NOT include 1<br>2. Clinically significant: tight CI | Width of CI: indicates the amount of variability and is a reflection of the sample size; also indicates clinical significance. |
| Odds ratio (OR) and relative risk (RR) | 1. OR >1: risk is greater in the exposed group<br>2. OR <1: risk is less in the exposed group<br>3. OR = 1: no difference | The larger the OR, the stronger the association between the exposure and disease. |
| Number needed to treat (NNT) (1/ARR) | The lower the number, the more effective the treatment is to bring about a significant effect change. | For example, for every 100 people treated, five deaths are avoided. Whenever NNT is considered, we must specify the follow-up period over which the difference was observed and the unfavorable outcome that was avoided. |
| Number needed to harm (NNH) | The higher this number is, the safer the treatment is before it causes harm. | For example, we treated 500 subjects before one was harmed. |
| Absolute risk reduction (ARR) | (CER – EER) | – |
| Relative risk reduction (RRR) | 100-RR%<br>(CER – EER)/CER | – |

CER, control event rate; EER, experimental event rate.

that half as many patients in the active group have an event at any point in time compared with placebo, again proportionately.

- Hazard ratios are not only used to determine survival but also to describe how many people can reach a certain point in time without experiencing a hazard or event other than death (e.g., having a heart attack).

Statistics used in research tend to be complex and often require the expertise of a statistician to not only interpret the data but also aid in choosing the type of testing used to validate data. Therefore, to not fully understand it at its core is normal and only expected. Hopefully, this chapter dove into the most commonly used statistical methods in medical research. Table 4.5 summarizes additional concepts not only used in the medial literature but also in medical examinations.

References

1. Swinscow TDV, Campbell MJ. *Statistics at Square One.* London: BMJ Books; 2002.

2. Lawless JF. *Statistical Models and Methods for Lifetime Data.* New York: John Wiley & Sons; 1982.

3. Armitage P, Berry G, Matthews JNS. *Statistical Methods in Medical Research.* 4th ed. Oxford, UK: Blackwell Science; 2002.

4. Lang TA, Secic M. *How to Report Statistics in Medicine: Annotated Guidelines for Authors, Editors, and Reviewers.* Philadelphia: American College of Physicians; 1997.

5. Fischer JE, Bachman LM, Jaeschke R. A readers' guide to the interpretation of diagnostic test properties: clinical example of sepsis. *Intensive Care Med.* 2003; 29:1043-1051.

6. Indrayan A, Bansal AK. The methods of survival analysis for clinicians. *Indian Pediatr.* 2010;47(9):743-748.

7. Bewick V, Cheek L, Ball J. Statistics review 12: survival analysis. *Crit Care.* 2004; 8(5):389-394.

8. Akobeng AK. Understanding diagnostic tests 3: Receiver operating characteristic curves. *Acta Paediatr.* 2007;96(5):644-647.

9. Ried K. Interpreting and understanding meta-analysis graphs—a practical guide. *Aust Fam Physicia*n. 2006;35(8):635-638.

10. Spruance SL, Reid JE, Grace M, Samore M. Hazard ratio in clinical trials. *Antimicrob Agents Chemother.* 2004;48(8):2787-2792.

# 5

# HOW TO PLAN RESEARCH

## APPROACH TO A RESEARCH QUESTION

Asking focused questions based on practical needs is one of the most effective ways to identify what research is relevant. Because limited time is available in medical school and residency for research, it is important to approach a research project in a systematic and realistic manner. Figure 5.1 details a realistic approach to a research project. The timeline certainly depends on the type of research being conducted. It is always important to have realistic goals in completing a research project because numerous factors such as Institutional Review Board (IRB) approval and statistical analysis require timeful consideration. The general approach to a research question should begin at least 2 to 3 months before the intended start date of the project. The study type that can best answer the particular research question at hand must be determined not only on a purely scientific basis, but also in view of the available financial resources, staffing, and practical feasibility (organization, medical prerequisites, number of patients, etc.).[1] A quick and easy way to organize your ideas and research question is to remember the 4 D's: Define, Design, Data Collection, and Deduction (Fig. 5.1). The general approach to a research question should begin at least 2–3 months before the intended start date of the project (Fig. 5.2).[2] In order to efficiently and effectively organize your project, one should consider the following:

1. Identification of a mentor: Identifying a mentor is the first step in initiation of a research project. A mentor supervises the project and makes sure that the question is focused and all prerequisite documentation is completed. The mentor also guides you as to whether your project is feasible given the allotted time.

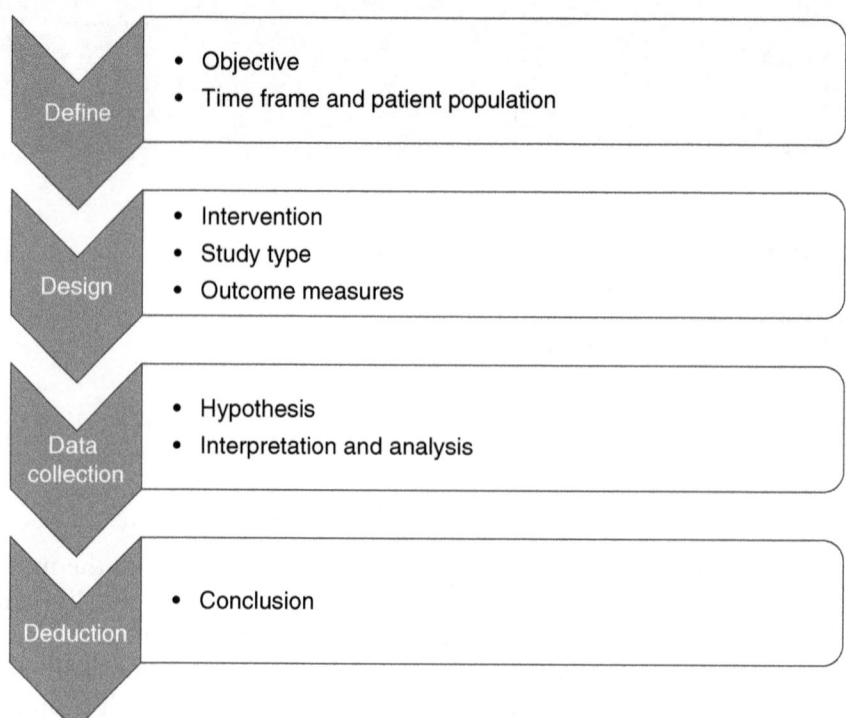

**FIGURE 5.1** Organizing a research question. The 4Ds of organizing a research question are define, design, data collection, and deduction.

2. Research required module completion or Collaborative Institutional Training Initiative (CITI) certification: Depending on the type of research you are conducting (human vs. animal), some programs require that you complete certain research modules that may require 1 or 2 days. Examples include the CITI that provides research ethics training modules. Make sure you check with your institution on whether certain modules are required.

3. Research question: This is centered around the PICO(T) paradigm.

4. Literature review: Give yourself ample time to conduct an extensive literature search on your topic to identify what clinical knowledge exists regarding your topic and what clinical knowledge lacks. This helps you build a stronger study.

5. Proposal: Construct a proposal of your research question according to Figure 5.3.

6. IRB: Make sure that you contact the Institutional Review Board (IRB) at your institution to inquire about timelines for submission.

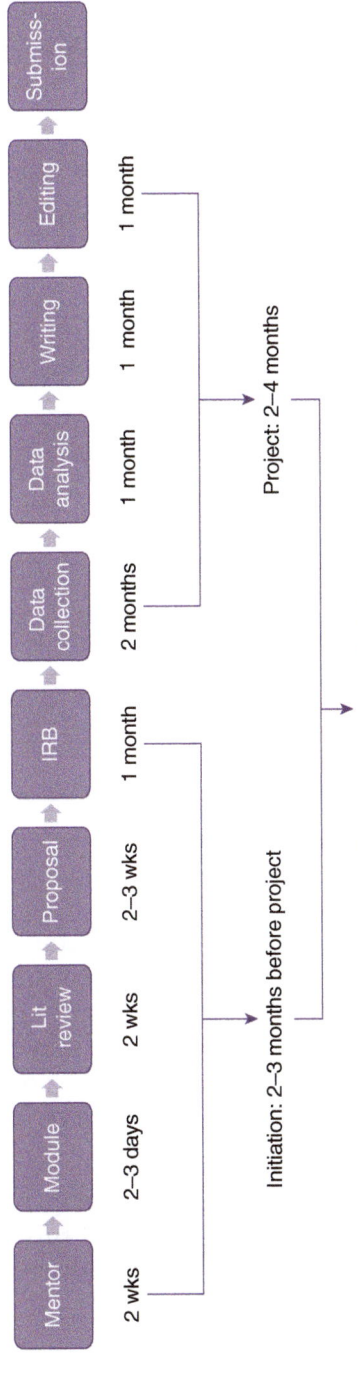

**FIGURE 5.2** Research project timeline.

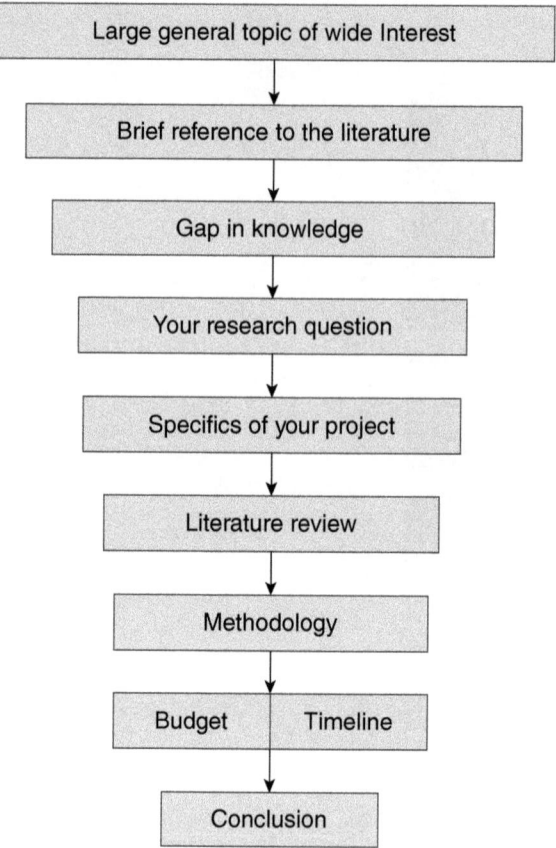

**FIGURE 5.3** The research proposal algorithm. This is a quick and fast way to start a research proposal.

An application is usually required that is lengthy and requires ample time. Certain IRBs meet at certain times during the month and have certain submission deadlines. It is also important to note that even after the IRB reviews your proposal, you may need to edit some things and resubmit it; therefore, make sure you give this at least 2 months in advance of initiating your project.

7. Data collection: The time frame for this part of your project heavily depends on what type of project you are pursing. Whether it is a retrospective chart review, cross-sectional survey, or cohort, data collection usually takes at least 1 or 2 months.

8. Data analysis: After data have been collected, it requires organization into tables or Excel spreadsheets with statistical analysis. In case a statistician is available, he or she should be contacted in advance in order to get a sense of his or her time framework.

9. **Writing:** After all the data have been collected and analyzed, writing is usually the easiest step. However, this may also require you to construct tables, figures, and graphs that may be time-consuming.

10. **Editing:** After the first draft is completed, it should be reviewed with your mentor and any other additional pertinent personnel.

11. **Submission:** This is the easiest step! It is important, however, to review the journal requirements for submission because they tend to have specific requirements for text and images that need to be met (Fig. 5.4).

A good way to look at planning of your project is the pie graph (Fig. 5.5) that depicts the research design project. The majority of your time (60%) should be spent planning the study. This includes defining the questions, variables, methods, designs, sampling plan, and methods of data collection. This is followed by executing the study by conducting it and collecting the data (10% of your time). Finally, it should

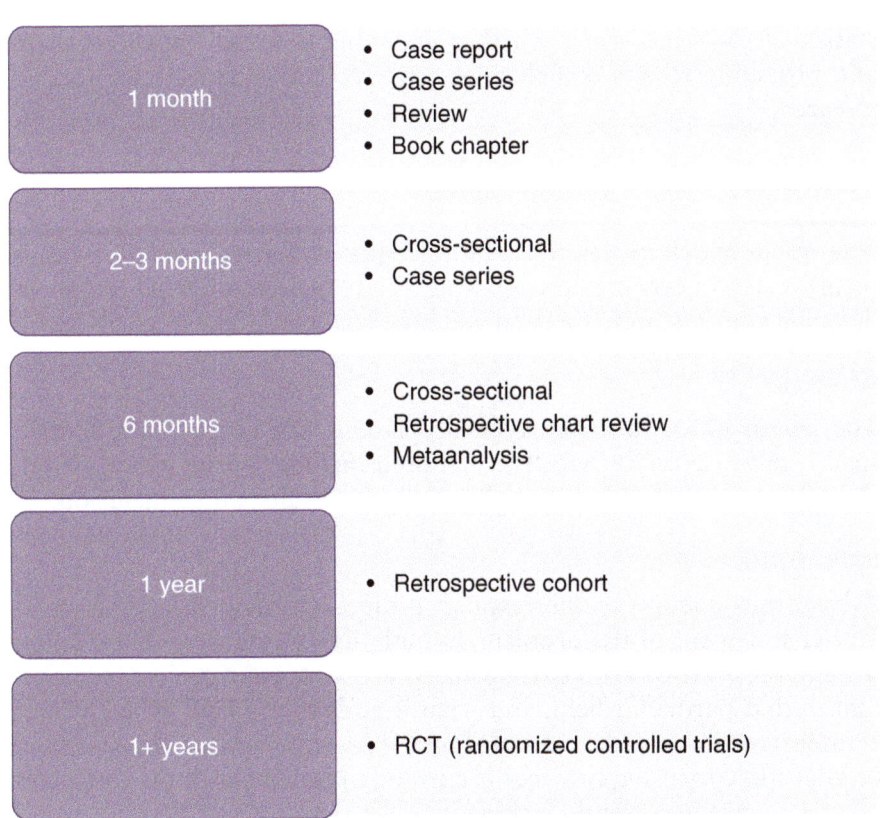

**FIGURE 5.4** Time-conscience research projects.

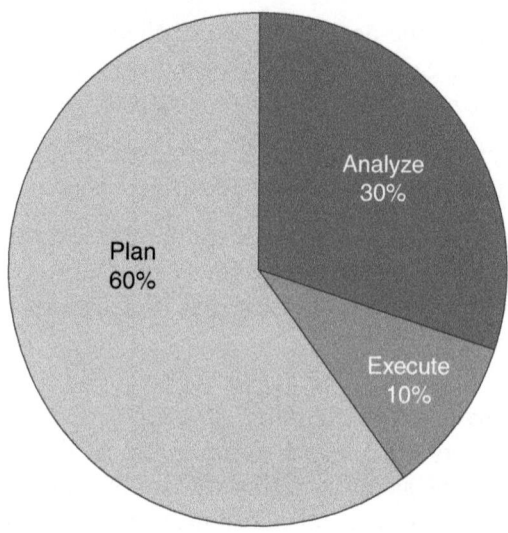

**FIGURE 5.5** The research design process.

be concluded by analysis of the data (30% of your time) by means of statistical tools; assessing whether your question has been answered; and providing results, conclusions, and recommendations for further research.[3,4]

## THE RESEARCH PROPOSAL

After the research question has been identified, the research proposal is the next step in organizing your work. The research proposal is a paper detailing your research question and how you would like to go about it.[5]

### Abstract

The length of the abstract typically should not exceed one double-spaced page (200–300 words). It should include a brief introduction, the aims or objective of the study, methods, results, and conclusion.

### Introduction

A brief introduction to the research project is provided leading up to a brief statement of the problem, hypothesis, or question. This should include the aims or objectives of the study, why your project is important in that particular field, and what it adds to the field. Therefore, it is important to provide a detailed and focused review of the literature on that topic focusing on what is currently known about the topic and what evidence is currently lacking.

## Methods

The methods section should include information regarding your population, including the sample size you wish to include in each arm and inclusion and exclusion criteria. Details regarding the procedure of the study should include how you wish to obtain the information, including data collection methods and instruments, as well as which variable you intend on measuring. Data analysis methods should specify how you wish to analyze the data with respect to statistical measures, as well as mechanisms to ensure the quality of the study, including bias, safety, and ethical considerations, and controlling for confounding factors.

## Budget

A research proposal should include an estimate to the budget of the study, including finances associated with data collection and data analysis.

## Appendices

The appendix of the research proposal should include not only the references but also copies of questionnaires, consent forms, and other important documentation that you anticipate using in your study (Fig. 5.3).

## APPLICATION OF A RESEARCH QUESTION

Let us assume that you are interested in exploring medical students' knowledge with respect to drinking caffeinated beverages. Your research question would be: Is the regular consumption of caffeinated beverages associated with improved academic performance among medical students? Table 5.1 documents different ways to implement this research question based on the time available and the research design you wish to used. First identify your research question via PICO(T):

Population: U.S. medical students (Med 1-4)

Intervention: Caffeinated beverages (coffee vs. sodas). Define type: are your measuring coffee or sodas? Define amount: more than 4 cups of coffee per week for the past year versus more than 4 cans of soda per week for 1 year.

Comparison: Noncaffeinated beverages

Outcome: Academic performance (USMLE scores, Shelf exam scores, memory, vigilance, concentration, fatigue scores)

**TABLE 5.1** Application of a Research Question: Medical Students' Knowledge and Caffeinated Beverages.

| Study Type | Description | Methods | Positives | Negatives |
|---|---|---|---|---|
| Case Control | To study a **rare account:** the association between regular caffeine consumption and acceptance in highly selective residencies | **Cases:** Fourth year medical students accepted to residency in "highly selective specialty X" **Control:** Fourth year medical students who applied but did not get in **Predictor:** Self-reported | Establishes association (odds ratio), inexpensive, efficient, generates hypotheses | Cannot determine incidence or prevalence, selection bias, recall bias |
| Cohort | The association of USMLE scores in medical students consuming caffeinated beverages | **Population:** All entering medical students **Method:** Surveyed regarding caffeine consumption; updates annually for 4 years to record changes in consumption **Outcomes:** USMLE Step 1 score, USMLE Step 2 score, match in first choice residency | Establishes incidence (relative risk) | Loss to follow-up, time-consuming, expensive |
| Cross-sectional | The prevalence of caffeine consumption in medical students with high USMLE scores | A questionnaire administered to students registering for USMLE 1 and asking them regarding caffeine consumption | Study prevalence, fast and inexpensive, no waiting, no loss to follow-up, can study associations | Cannot determine causality, cannot study rare outcomes |
| Randomized controlled trial (RCT) | An RCT of daily caffeine consumption among entering medical students | Randomized to daily consumption of Red Bull vs. daily consumption of placebo **Outcomes:** USMLE Step 1 score, USMLE Step 2 score, match in first choice residency | Can determine causality, relative risk, intention to treat analysis | Loss to follow-up, expensive, time-consuming |

References

1. Röhrig B, du Prel JB, Wachtlin D, Blettner M. Types of study in medical research. Part 3 of a series on evaluation of scientific publications. *Dtsch Arztebl Int.* 2009; 106(15):262-268.

2. Bickman L, Rog DJ. *Applied Research Design, A Practical Approach.* Sage; 1997.

3. Hartung DM, Touchette D. Overview of clinical research design. *Am J Health-Syst Pharm.* 2009;66:398-408.

4. Machin D, Campbell MJ: *Design of Studies for Medical Research.* Chichester, UK: Wiley; 2005;1-286.

5. Röhrig B, du Prel JB, Blettner M. Study design in medical research. Part 2 of a series on the evaluation of scientific publications. *Dtsch Arztebl Int.* 2009;106(11):184-189.

# 6

# HOW TO ORGANIZE RESEARCH

## COLLECTING DATA

The first step in organizing and collecting your data is to decide what exactly you want to collect. Most research projects have a primary and secondary end point, which formulate the basis for data collection. It is important, however, to collect other ancillary data that may elicit important points relevant to your research. One of the easiest and most important sets of data to collect is demographic data. This not only provides a way to distinguish whether there are differences among age groups, race, and gender but also provides an important basis for describing the population selected. This is critical because it is vital to show that the sample that you started out with is similar in these potential confounding aspects, which decreases the risk of biases. Similarly, it is important to collect data on other confounding factors that you may think might affect the result of your study. Examples include patients who were already taking certain medications, comorbid conditions, smoking status, and so on. After you decide what parameters you want to collect, the next step is organizing these data into a form feasible for analysis.

## DATA STORAGE AND PROTECTION

When patient information is collected, it is important to contain this information in a safe and secure manner. This is not only important for avoiding bias but for also protecting patient information. This can be achieved by de-identifying the data and assigning codes to each subject. Additionally, storing it in an encrypted and password protected computer is also essential.

## DATA COLLECTION

Whether your research study is descriptive or experiential, the easiest way to collect and organize data is in Excel. Excel is a good tool for calculations, simple descriptive statistics creating graphs, charts, and diagrams and organizing lists.[1]

A few tips:

1. The coding scheme: When entering and analyzing data, it is easiest to work with numbers. To do this, a number is assigned to each possible response option. For example male = 1; female = 2. It is important to go over the coding system with your principal investigator and a statistician to determine the best coding system for your data in order to facilitate analysis.

2. How missing data are represented: Never use zero to indicate missing data. Zero is especially likely to be misinterpreted as an actual value rather than as missing data.

3. Use a separate column for each parameter.

4. Data analysis: The majority of the data analysis should be discussed with a statistician. Depending on what type of information you wish to extract from the data, the statistician will be able to advise you

**TABLE 6.1** Simple Statistical Formulas in Excel.

| Calculate | Using the Function/ Formula | Example |
|---|---|---|
| The number of questionnaires completed | ROWS | =ROWS(B2:B7) |
| The average scores of those who responded | AVERAGE | =AVERAGE (B2:B7) |
| The lowest score given as an answer | MIN | =MIN(B2:B7) |
| The highest score given as an answer | MAX | =MAX(B2:B7) |
| The number of respondents who gave a specific answer | COUNTIF | =COUNTIF(B2:B7) |
| The most frequently occurring score | MEDIAN | =MEDIAN(B2:B7) |
| The variability of scores | STANDARD DEVIATION | =STDEV(B2:B7) |

**TABLE 6.2** Statistical Tests Used in Excel.

| Test | Purpose |
| --- | --- |
| Two-sample *t*-test | To check whether the two treatment groups differ on the values of either X or Y |
| Paired *t*-test | To test whether the difference between two measurements on the same subject are significantly different from 0 |
| Chi-square | To test for a relationship between treatment and outcome |
| Pivot tables | To obtain simple frequencies and cross-tabulations |
| Analysis of variance (ANOVA) | To test the means of two groups and determine if the difference between them is statistically significant |
| Linear regression | To determine linear relationships between two or more variables; regression analysis works by fitting a line that best describes the relationship |

as what the best statistical tool to use. You can also conduct your own preliminary analysis by using Excel. In Excel, you can calculate averages, medians, and simple *t*-tests that can be useful in describing demographic data. Additionally, for more experienced Excel users, pivot tables serve as a vital tool to extract certain types of data. Pivot tables can be used as an alternate way to create frequency distributions, although they cannot be used for multiple response questions. They can also be used to create cross-tabulations of data. For example, in a study of the effect of drug A and placebo in allergic rhinitis, you may wish to know how many subjects were taking drug A and had decreased number of sneezes. It allows one to pull or extract tied data (Tables 6.1 and 6.2).

Reference

1. Elliott AC, Hynan LS, Reisch JS, Smith JP. Preparing data for analysis using Microsoft Excel. *J Investig Med.* 2006;54(6):334-341.

# 7

# HOW TO PRESENT YOUR RESEARCH

*Abstracts, posters, and presentations*

## ABSTRACTS

Abstracts are typically condensed research summaries embodied in a mere 300 to 400 words. Mastering the skill of writing an abstract will increase the probability of selection at a scientific program.[1]

### Outline of an Abstract[2]

1. Title: Summarizes abstract and includes authors and affiliations

2. Introduction: Summarizes the clinical problem (two to three sentences)

3. Methods: Describes study design, setting, sample and control selection, outcome measures, and statistical analysis

4. Results: Begins with a description of the study sample, controls, and exclusions and then lists the frequencies of the most frequent outcomes; describes comparisons of outcomes between and among groups

5. Conclusion: Summarizes conclusions and implications of study

## POSTERS

1. Poster planning: Know the rules: Each conference or meeting has a specific set of requirements for poster size, organization, and display specifications. It is important to review the size of the board that will hold the poster in order to determine size of the poster.

2. Poster production: Posters should follow the general IMRAD format:
   - Introduction: Includes background information summarizing current knowledge in the area, gaps in knowledge, and the purpose of study in addressing that gap

- **Methods:** Includes research design, inclusion and exclusion criteria for patients, outcome variables, and methods of statistical analysis
- **Results:** Includes frequencies of the most important outcome variables, graphs, and tables
- **Discussion:** Includes the study conclusion, implications, and limitations

Clinical vignette posters follow the ICD format:

- **Introduction:** Describes context of the case and whether it has been reported in the literature before
- **Case description:** Describes in sequence the patient's history, physical examination findings, ancillary studies, treated options, and patient's progress and outcome
- **Discussion:** Reviews why certain decisions have been made, extracts a lesson from the case, or describes a new presentation of a particular pathologic phenomenon

Tips for poster content:

1. Proofread: Make sure there are no grammatical or syntax errors, that everyone's name is spelled correctly, and that you include the name and location of your institution and whether your project was funded by anyone.

2. Include titles, authors, institutional affiliations, and funding sources.

3. Avoid clutter: Each section should be concise and clear with color, lines, boxes, and arrows used to emphasize important points.

4. For research posters: Introduction, methods, results and discussion (IMRAD)

5. For clinical vignettes: Introduction, case description, and discussion (ICD)

6. Logical sequence of information flow (left to right and top to bottom)

Tips for poster appearance:

1. Poster meets size restrictions of the scientific program.

2. Abstract is on the poster (if required).

3. Major heading can be read from 3 to 5 feet away.

4. Text and figures can be read from 2 to 4 feet away.

5. Graphs and figures can be read from 2 to 3 feet away.

6. Font is similar throughout (no more than three font sizes are used throughout: poster title, section title, text).

7. Overall content can be absorbed in 10 minutes or less.

## Poster Judging Criteria

1. Originality: How original is the concept presented in this poster? Or how original is the new approach to an old problem?

2. Significance: How significant are the poster's conclusions in increasing understanding of a disease process or in improving the diagnosis or treatment of a disease state?

3. Presentation: How logical are the ideas presented in this poster? How interesting is the manner of presentation?

4. Methods: If applicable, how suitable is the research design for the stated objectives, and how appropriate are any statistical techniques applied?

5. Visual impact: How effective is this poster visually? How valuable is each figure and graph in furthering viewers' understanding of the research subject?

6. Interview: How knowledgeable and conversant is the presenting author with the research presented in the poster?

## Poster Tutorial

- Know the size requirement of your poster.
- Know the size of the board where you will hang your poster.
- Helpful tip: Create an A4 size of your poster with your contact information so you may be able to hand it to any of your interested audience (Table 7.1).

Remember:

1. Font sizes:[3,4]

Title: 80 to 100 pt (readable from 25 ft away); average, 85 pt
Authors: 56 pt
Section Headings: 35 to 70 pt; average, 36 pt
Text: 25 to 35 pt (readable from 4 to 6 ft away); average, 25 pt
Captions: 18 pt
To be legible from 6 feet, use 30 pt
To be legible from 10 feet, use 48 pt
To be legible from 12 feet, use 60 pt
To be legible from 14 feet, use 72 pt

**TABLE 7.1** Translating PowerPoint to a Poster.[5]

| Page setup | File>Page Set-up>Custom>Poster Size<br>PowerPoint will not let you use a custom page size that is larger than 56 inches. To work around this limitation, you'll need to set up your file to a smaller proportionate scale. |
|---|---|
| Font sizes | 1. Title: 84 pt (96 pt is better)<br>2. Authors: 42 pt<br>3. Section headings: 30 pt (48 pt is better)<br>4. Text: 28 pt (32 pt is better)<br>5. Literature cites and acknowledgement: 18 to 20 pt<br>6. Font: Times New Roman or Arial |
| Images and graphics | 1. For printing, your images should be about 300 dpi.<br>2. Inserting a picture or graphic as a file as opposed to TIF provides the best format for printing high-quality images. You can always create a JPEG image later from your TIF. (JPEG is the best choice for color photos on the Internet.)<br>3. Copy the graph: Edit menu>Paste Special>>Picture (Enhanced Metafile)<br>4. Items pasted as a **Microsoft Office Graphic Object** will insert as a graphic object that can be edited in PowerPoint.<br>5. Items pasted as a picture cannot be edited; items pasted as an enhanced metafile cannot be edited in their native applications. |
| Moving objects | Move objects to *exactly* where you want them. If you want to place an object, such as an arrow, picture, or text box, very precisely, hold down Alt while you move the object around with the mouse. It gives you a much freer range of motion. |

2. Font: Times New Roman or Arial

3. Proportional sizes (PowerPoint vs. final poster)

PowerPoint: $48 \times 24$ or a $1 \times 2$ ratio

Therefore can be printed as $18 \times 36$ or $36 \times 72$

Problem: If you want to print a different aspect ratio than what is set up your PowerPoint:

Example: Desired poster dimensions: $36 \times 54$, PowerPoint page set up: $48 \times 24$

→ Resize your PowerPoint file

4. How will my poster look when it is printed? For example: Consider a PowerPoint page setup size of 24″ by 32″ and a desired print size of 42″ by 56″.

- Take the vertical dimension of the print size and divide it by the vertical dimension of the page setup size in your PowerPoint: $42 \div 24 = 1.75$
- Multiply it by 100 to get your viewing percentage: $1.75 * 100 = 175\%$

Now simply enter that percentage into the zoom percentage box.

- Examine the various images, graphs, headings, and text boxes of your poster while standing a few feet from your monitor at this zoomed in percentage to get a good feel for whether the quality and sizing will work well on your final printed poster.

5. Changing page size with existing content:

Select everything on your slide by pressing Ctrl + A.
Cut everything from your slide by pressing Ctrl + X.
Go to the Design tab, select Page Setup, and change the size.
Paste all of the items back on the slide by pressing Ctrl + V.
At this point, you will most likely have a lot of extra space on your slide or have a lot of your content hanging off of the slide boundaries.

### Poster Handout

Print a mini-sized version of your poster with your contact information on the back. This provides a little more detail about your work and also achieves the important goal of sending your audience away with your work and your name in hand.

## POWERPOINT PRESENTATIONS

A. Logistics
- Disclosures: Always include a slide at the beginning stating you have no disclosures that may affect the validity and reliability of your presentation.
- Time: One of the greatest obstacles is the strict time limit. Therefore, if allotted only 15 minutes for the presentation, plan and practice your presentation as if you have only 10 to 12 minutes. This gives you time in case you get nervous or forget something and for audience Q&A.
- Acknowledgements: Acknowledge sources of support and research assistance at the end of your presentation as a courtesy to all those who helped you.

B. Presentation skills
- First, be sure to leave the title slide up long enough for your audience to read it: It allows your audience to read your title and your name.

- Make sure you have good transition sentences between each slide.
- If you plan to use a laser pointer, practice with it but use it minimally; otherwise, it is too distracting.
- Know your material well!
  - Memorize as much of the presentation as possible.
  - Dress professionally.
  - Address your audience: Look at the audience, not at the screen. It is very tempting to read off your slides, but it is awful to watch. Read from your notes or the computer screen if you can get it facing the right way. The best method is to memorize certain notes you wish to include verbally as opposed to including them in the presentation.
- Answer the question: If a question is unexpected and you do not know how to answer it, you can say, "That is a very interesting question; however, we did not explore that in our study, or that was the limitation of the study."

C. Design
- Computer compatibility: If you use a Mac, make sure your theme uses Windows-safe fonts.
- Colors
  - A plain white background is classic. A plain black background looks great in a dark room and adds emphasis to your data because it appears with no border. Royal blue has also been used with much success with yellow and white headings.
  - Make sure colors are not too distracting and do not make the text illegible.
- Diagrams and images
  - Slides with only writing can be difficult to focus on. Use flow charts or concept maps where possible.
  - Every image, diagram, and graph should have a caption or annotation.
  - Images from other sources should be cited accurately.
- Graphs and charts
  - All graphs should look the same with the same color and layout.
  - Headings and legends should be consistently labeled.
  - Include error bars, and comparisons should have significant values.
  - Each experimental group should have a consistent color or format in all graphs.

- Text
  - Font: Choose a font that is easy to read such as Arial, Times New Roman or Courier.
  - Use the same typeface throughout your presentation.
  - If you are a Mac user, avoid fonts that do not go across platforms, such as Helvetica.
  - Spacing: 1.5 spacing so that the lines are easier to follow.
  - Size: Use a font that is about as large as the slide will accommodate; for example, title lines size 44, major text 32, and minor text 24.

D. Content
- Do not write full sentences on slides. They should be readable in one glance.
- Keep data on each slide to a minimum.
- Do not include anything that you are uncomfortable with on a slide.
- Your conclusion slide must be able to be read from the back of the room.

## GUIDELINES FOR WRITING A SCIENTIFIC PAPER[6]

The success for writing a good scientific paper lies in making sure it contains all the core elements. It is often a difficult task and requires ample time and numerous proofreads. A good rule of thumb is to write as if your paper will be read by a person who knows about the field in general but does not already know what you did. Before you write a scientific paper, read some scientific papers that have been written in the format of the paper you plan to use as well as in the field you wish to write about. It is critical to know the present literature surrounding the topic you wish to write about (Table 7.2).

1. Abstract: A succinct (one-paragraph) summary of the entire paper. The abstract should briefly describe the question posed in the paper, the methods used to answer this question, the results obtained, and the conclusions. It should be possible to determine the major points of a paper by reading the abstract. Although it is located at the beginning of the paper, it is easiest to write the abstract after the paper is completed.

2. Introduction
   - Describe the question tested by the experiments.
   - Explain why this is an interesting or important question.

**TABLE 7.2** Sections of a Scientific Paper.

| Experimental Process | Section of Paper |
|---|---|
| What did I do in a nutshell? | Abstract |
| What is the problem? | Introduction |
| How did I solve the problem? | Materials and Methods |
| What did I find out? | Results |
| What does it mean? | Discussion |
| Who helped me? | Acknowledgments (optional) |
| Whose work did I refer to? | Literature Cited |
| Extra information | Appendices (optional) |

- Describe the approach used.
- Briefly mention the conclusion of the paper.

3. Materials and methods: The Materials and Methods section should succinctly describe the techniques used. The details of a published protocol do not need to be reproduced in the text, but an appropriate reference should be cited or placed in a supplement appendix.
   - Population: Describe the population to be studied, inclusion and exclusion criteria, and how they were selected.
   - Design: The type of study used (double blind, randomized, prospective)
   - Collecting data: Describe the primary and secondary endpoints and how they will be collected.
   - Analyzing data: Statistical tools and methods used to analyze the data and who will be responsible for this task
   - Confidentiality and privacy: When applicable, this pertains to patient-sensitive information. You should mention whether patient identifiers will be coded and confidential.
   - Financial gain: It is important to mention whether your study was sponsored by a pharmaceutical company

4. Results: Begin each paragraph with an opening sentence that tells readers what question is being tested in the experiments described in that paragraph. When referring to a particular table or figure, they should be capitalized (e.g., Table 1, Figure 6). The text of the Results section should be succinct but should provide readers with

a summary of the results of each table or figure. Negative results are still results! If you did not get the anticipated results, it may mean your hypothesis was incorrect and needs to be reformulated or perhaps you have stumbled onto something unexpected that warrants further study.

5. Discussion: Do not simply restate the results; instead, explain your conclusions and interpretations of the Results section. How did your results compare with the expected results? What further predictions can be gleaned from the results? Remember, do not introduce new results into the discussion part. Important concepts to remember include:
   - Do your results provide answers to your testable hypotheses? If so, how do you interpret your findings?
   - Do your findings agree with what others have shown? If not, do they suggest an alternative explanation or perhaps an unforeseen design flaw in your experiment (or theirs)?
   - Given your conclusions, what is our new understanding of the problem you investigated and outlined in the Introduction?
   - If warranted, what would be the next step in your study (e.g., what experiments would you do next)?

## CONCLUSION: A FEW HELPFUL TIPS IN PRESENTING RESEARCH

1. Abbreviations: Define all abbreviations the first time they are used; then subsequently use the abbreviation.

2. Past, present, and future tense: Results described in your paper should be described in the past tense. Results from published papers should be described in the present tense.

3. Third versus first person: It is acceptable to use first person in scientific writing, but it should be used sparingly; reserve the use of first person for things that you want to emphasize that "you" uniquely did (i.e., not things that many others have done as well). Most text should be written in the third person to avoid sounding like an autobiographical account.

4. Appendices: An appendix contains information that is nonessential to understanding of the paper but may present information that further clarifies a point without burdening the body of the presentation. Examples of material included in appendices include raw data, extra images, figures, and tables.

## References

1. Pierson DJ. How to write an abstract that will be accepted for presentation at a national meeting. *Respir Care.* 2004;49(10):1206-1212.

2. Patrick Alguire. Guide to Preparing for the Abstract Competition. Retrived online from American College of physicians. http://www.acponline.org/residents_fellows/competitions/abstract/prepare/. Accessed 8/2012.

3. Poster Tutorial. Retrieved online from: http://www.makesigns.com/tutorials/. Retrieved 8/2012.

4. Davis M. Poster presentations. In: *Scientific Papers and Presentations.* Revised ed. Burlington, MA: Academic Press; 2005:181-204.

5. Gosling PJ. *Scientist's Guide to Poster Presentations.* New York: Kluwer Academic/Plenum Press; 1999.

6. Day R. *How to Write and Publish a Scientific Paper.* 5th ed. Orynx Press, Phoenix AZ; 1998.

# 8

# DECIPHERING DIFFERENT RESEARCH DOMAINS

To understand and conduct research, sometimes it is easier to categorize it into its underlying domains: diagnosis, etiology, therapy, and prognosis studies. This chapter explores the best kind of evidence and studies used to explore each domain; discusses how to formulate a well-built PICOS question based on that domain, how to appraise a study, and what questions to ask based on the domain; and finally covers the most common statistical tools used in each domain. Using this categorization method, it allows for more comprehensive knowledge of research and a better understanding of how to conduct research.

## THE BEST EVIDENCE

One of the steps in practicing evidence-based medicine involves accessing the clinical literature in order to assess the evidence. Depending on the type of study, different research designs can either heighten or subdue the level of evidence behind that study. For example, a double-blind, randomized, controlled trial about the comparison of intranasal steroids versus placebo in the treatment of allergic rhinitis would have a higher level of evidence than a case-control trial or a nonrandomized, noncontrolled, prospective trial. The data extracted from a double-blind, randomized, controlled trial hold more power than data extracted from a noncontrolled, nonrandomized trial primarily because of elements of validity, reproducibility, and applicability to the general population. Table 8.1 depicts the best research designs with the highest levels of evidence for each study domain.

## THE PICOS QUESTION

Similar to how there are better research designs tailored to each research domain, one should tailor the PICO question according to the type of research design. When dealing with diagnosis-based studies,

**TABLE 8.1** The Best Evidence for Each Research Domain.

| Domain | Evidence |
|---|---|
| Diagnosis | Systematic review of prospective cohort studies or cross-sectional studies with blind comparison with the diagnostic gold standard |
| Eitology, cause, and harm | Etiology and therapy studies: RCT or systemic reviews<br>Causation: Retrospective case-control studies, prospective cohorts |
| Therapy and prevention | Double-blind, randomized, controlled or systemic review of such trials (meta-analysis)<br>Prospective controlled |
| Prognosis | Systemic review of prospective cohorts |

RCT, randomized, controlled trial.

the questions to be asked regarding the population are: What are the characteristics of the patient, and what is the condition that might be present? This is in contrast to the question being asked regarding the population in a therapy-based study: How would I describe a group of patients similar to mine? This shows how different and unique the PICO system of asking questions is depending on the type of study. If you are conducting a study on a specific diagnostic test, your question pertaining to your population should focus around whether specific characteristics are found in that patient that make that condition present. This is compared with a therapy-based study in which the question surrounding the population should be focused more toward making sure that both groups are as similar as possible to avoid bias (Table 8.2).

## THE CLINICAL APPRAISAL

In previous chapters, the approach to critically appraising journal articles has been discussed. Therefore, this shall not be dealt with in this chapter. However, one should keep in mind certain questions when dealing with certain domain-specific articles.

### A. Questions You Should Ask in a Diagnostic Study
**Are the results valid?**

- Was there an independent blind comparison with a reference standard?
- Is reference standard used acceptable?

**TABLE 8.2** PICO Questions for Each Type of Research Domain.

| PICOS | Studies | | | |
|---|---|---|---|---|
| | Diagnosis | Etiology, Causation, and Harm | Therapy | Prognosis |
| Population and patient | What are the characteristics of the patients? What is the condition that may be present? | How would I describe a group of patients similar to mine? | How would I describe a group of patients similar to mine (e.g., condition, age, gender, )? | How would I describe a cohort of patients similar to mine? |
| Intervention | Which diagnostic test am I considering? | Which main exposure am I considering? | Which main or new intervention am I considering? | Which main prognostic factor am I considering? |
| Comparison | What is the diagnostic gold standard? | What is the main alternative to compare with the exposure? | What is the alternative to compare with the intervention (e.g., placebo, standard of care)? | What is the comparison group, if any? |
| Outcome | How likely is the test to predict or rule out this condition? | How is the incidence or prevalence of the condition in this group affected by this exposure? | What can I hope to accomplish, measure, improve, or affect? | What disease progression can be expected? |
| Study design | What study design would provide the best level of evidence for this question? | | | |

- Were both reference standard and test applied to all patients?
- Did the patient sample include an appropriate spectrum of patients to whom the test will be applied?
- Did the results of the test being evaluated influence the decision to perform the reference standard ("verification" or "workup" bias)?

- Were the test's methods described clearly enough to permit replication?
  - Preparation of patient?
  - Performance of test?
  - Analysis and interpretation of results?

## What are the likelihood ratios for the test results?

- What are the likelihood ratios for the test results?

## Will the results help me care for my patients?

- Will the test be reproducible and well interpreted in my practice setting?
- Are the results applicable to my patients?
  - Similar distribution of disease severity?
  - Similar distribution of competing diseases?
  - Compelling reasons why the results should not be applied?
- Will the test results change my management?
  - Test and treatment thresholds?
  - High or low likelihood ratios?
- Will my patients be better off because of the test?
  - Is target disorder dangerous if left undiagnosed?
  - Is test risk acceptable?
  - Does effective treatment exist?
- Will information from test lead to change of management beneficial to patient?


## B. Questions You Should Ask in an Etiology Study

## Are the results valid?

- Except for the exposure under study, were the compared groups similar to each other?
  - Randomized, controlled trial (RCT), cohort, case control?
  - Other known prognosis factors similar or adjusted for?
- Were the outcomes and exposures measured in the same way in the compared groups?
  - Recall bias? Interviewer bias?
  - Exposure opportunity similar?
- Was follow-up sufficiently long and complete?
  - Reasons for incomplete follow-up?
  - Risk factors similar in those lost and not lost to follow-up?

- Is the temporal relationship correct?
  - Exposure preceded outcome?
- Is there a dose–response gradient?
  - Risk of outcome increases with quantity or duration of exposure?

**What are the results?**

- How strong is the association between exposure and outcome?
  - Relative risk or odds ratio?
- How precise is the estimate of risk?
  - Confidence intervals?

**Will the results help me care for my patients?**

- Are the results applicable to my patients?
  - Patients similar for demographics, morbidity, and other prognostic factors?
  - Are treatments and exposures similar?
- What is the magnitude of the risk?
  - Absolute risk increase (and its reciprocal)?
- Should I attempt to stop the exposure?
  - Strength of evidence?
  - Magnitude of risk?
  - Adverse effects of reducing exposure?

## C. Questions You Should Ask in a Therapy Study

**Are the results valid?**

- Was the assignment of patients to treatment randomized?
- Were all patients who entered the trial properly accounted for and attributed at its conclusion?
  - Was follow-up complete?
  - Were patients analyzed in the groups to which they were randomized ?
  - Intention to treat analysis?
- Were patients, their clinicians, and study personnel "blind" to the treatment allocation?
- Were the groups similar at the start of the trial?
  - Baseline prognostic factors (demographics, comorbidity, disease severity, other known confounders) balanced?
  - If different, were these adjusted for?

- Aside from the experimental intervention, were the groups treated equally? What about
  - Cointerventions?
  - Contamination?
  - Compliance?

## What are the results?

- How large is the treatment effect?
  - Absolute risk reduction?
  - Relative risk reduction?
- Did the study have a sufficiently large sample size?
- How precise is the estimate of the treatment effect?
  - Confidence intervals?

## Will the results help me care for my patient?

- Can the results be applied to my patients?
  - Patients similar for demographics, severity, comorbidity, and other prognostic factors?
  - Compelling reason why they should not be applied?
- Were all clinically relevant outcomes considered?
- Are substitute endpoints valid?
- Are the benefits worth the harms and costs?
  - NNT (number needed to treat) for different outcomes?

## D. Questions You Should Ask in a Study of Prognosis

## Are the results valid?

- Was there a representative and well-defined sample of patients at a similar point in the course of disease?
  - Inclusion and exclusion criteria?
  - Selection bias?
  - Stage of disease?
- Was follow-up sufficiently long and complete?
  - Reasons for incomplete follow-up?
  - Prognostic factors similar for patients lost and not lost to follow-up?
- Were objective and unbiased outcome criteria used?
  - Outcomes defined at start of study?
  - Investigators "blind" to prognostic factors?
- Was there adjustment for important prognostic factors?

## What are the results?

- How likely are the outcomes over time? Survival curves (Kaplan–Meier)?
- How precise are the estimates of likelihood?
  - Confidence intervals?

## Will the results help me care for my patients?

- Were the study patients similar to my own?
  - Patients similar for demographics, severity, comorbidity, and other prognostic factors?
- Compelling reason why the results should not be applied?
- Will the results lead directly to selecting therapy?
- Are the results useful for reassuring patients?

### Notes on Understanding an Article on Prognosis

The prognosis of a disease refers to its possible outcomes and the likelihood that each one will occur.

A prognostic factor is a patient characteristic that can predict that patient's eventual outcome:

- Demographic: e.g., age
- Disease specific: e.g., tumor stage
- Comorbid: other conditions present

Prognostic results are the number of events that occur over time, expressed in:

- Absolute terms: e.g., 5-year survival rate
- Relative terms: e.g., risk from prognostic factor
- Survival curves: cumulative events over time

## THE STATISTICS

Whether the study at hand is a study focused on a treatment or diagnosis, it is helpful to know that certain statistical tools described in detail in previous chapters are in fact domain specific. This not only aids in understanding the complex interpretations of statistical tools but also aids in translating the data derived from this into practice. By knowing which statistical tools are used in which domain, one can not only develop a better understanding but also be able to create a well-constructed study (Table 8.3).

**TABLE 8.3** Statistical Tools Associated with Each Research Domain.

| | Studies | | | |
|---|---|---|---|---|
| | Diagnosis | Etiology, Causation, and Harm | Therapy | Prognosis |
| Statistical tests used | Sensitivity, specificity, positive and negative predictive value, likelihood ratio | Odds ratio, relative risk, attributable risk | Control event rate, experimental event rate, absolute risk, number needed to treat, relative risk, relative risk reduction | Absolute: survival rate Relative: risk from a prognostic factor Survival curve |

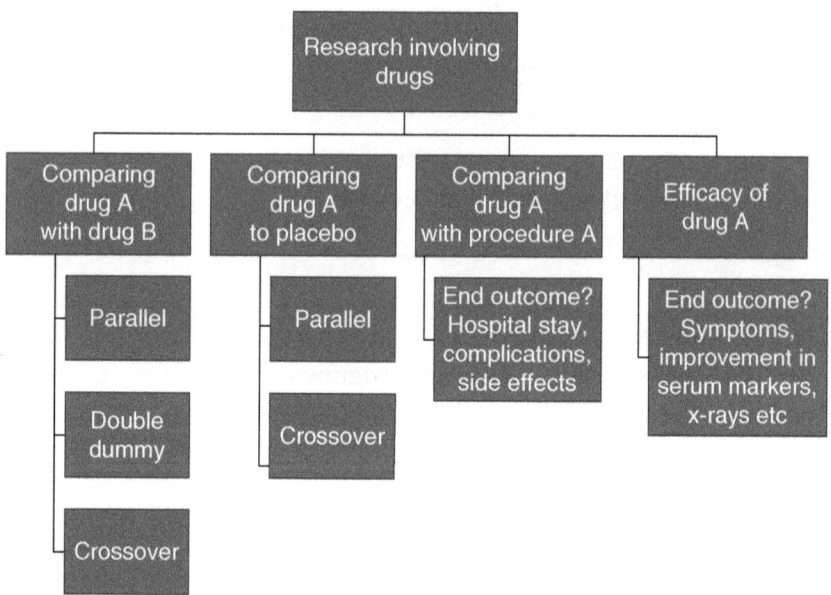

**FIGURE 8.1** Research involving drugs. This algorithm depicts different research methodologies involving research with treatment drugs.

## THE RESEARCH STUDY ALGORITHMS

1. **Research involving drugs:** After understanding how to decipher a specific study, it becomes easier to plan a research study. After understanding the different methodological designs, the way you ask your research question will help form your research study into numerous different designs. An example is provided in Figure 8.1 by illustrating the algorithm that is created in an attempt to design a research study involving therapy such as the use of certain drugs.

2. **Experimental research design algorithm:** Similar to the algorithm presented in Figure 8.1, if your question pertains to an experimental study, then based on your time frame, tools, budget, and research questions, you can construct different types of studies all with their own advantages and disadvantages (Fig. 8.2).

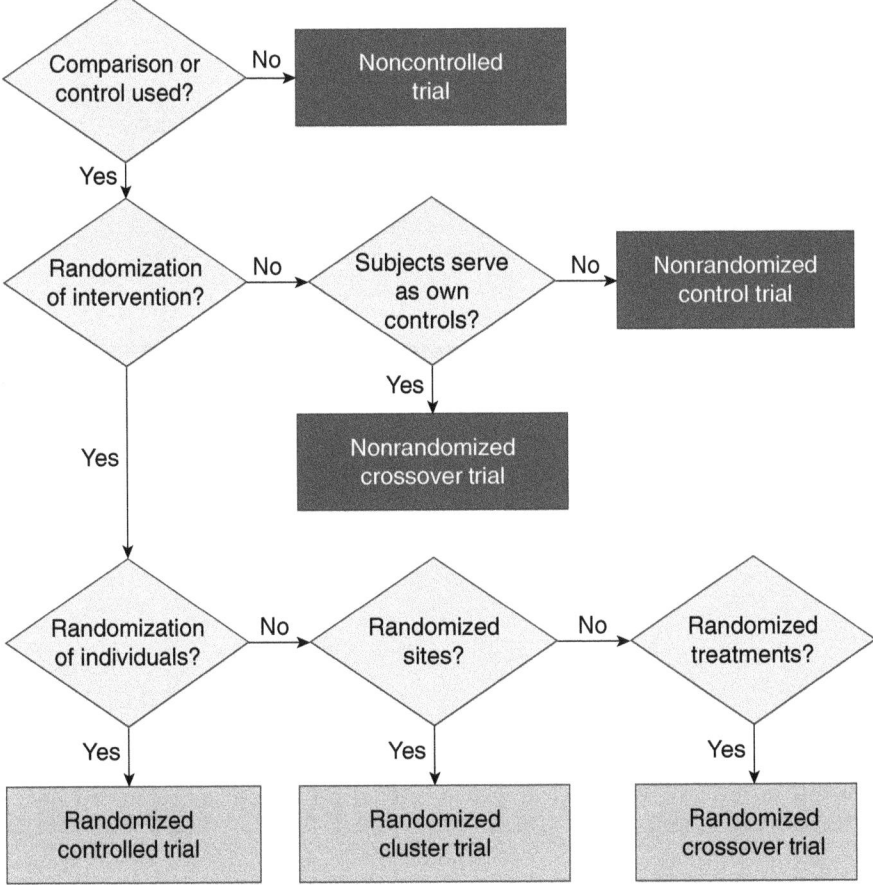

**FIGURE 8.2** Experimental research design algorithm: a general algorithm exploring experimental research design.

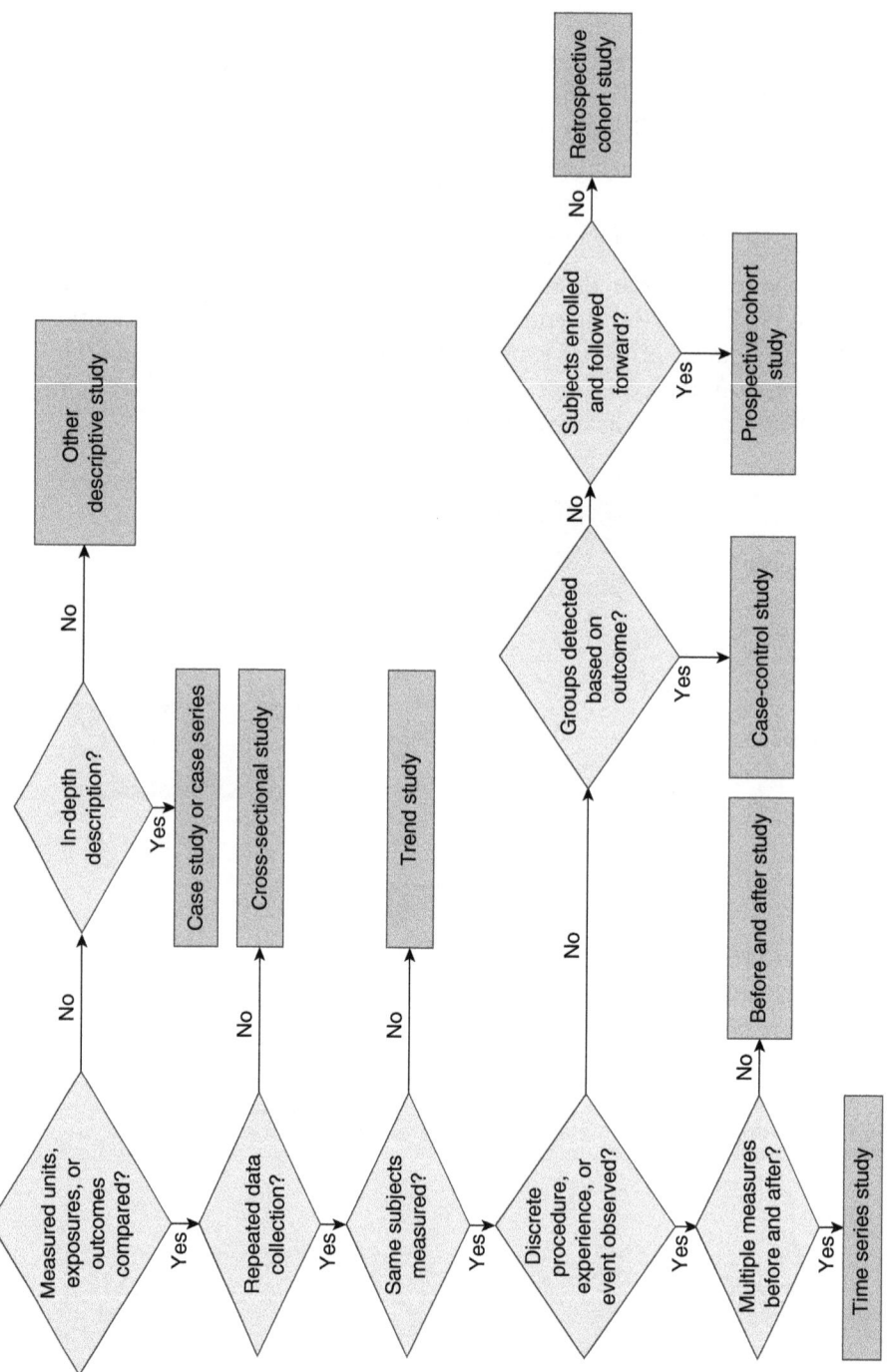

**FIGURE 8.3** Descriptive research design algorithm: a general algorithm exploring descriptive research design.

3. **Descriptive research design algorithm:** Descriptive research designs also follow similar patterns based on the investigators initial research question. Depending on how a research question is framed or posed and the tools available, one can construct a cross-sectional study, case study, or case-control study (Fig. 8.3).

# 9

# GLOSSARY OF TERMS

Absolute risk reduction (ARR): The arithmetic difference in risk or outcomes between treatment and control groups. Example: if the mortality rate is 30% in controls and 20% with treatment, the ARR is $30 - 20 = 10\%$.

Case-control study: A study in which subjects are selected on the basis of their outcomes and then exposures (treatments) are ascertained. For example, to assess the association between race and operative mortality, one might select all patients who died after open heart surgery in a given year and then select an equal number of patients who survived, matching on several variables other than race so as to equalize (control for) their distributions between the cases and noncases.

Categorical variable: A variable whose value ranges over categories, such as {red, green, blue}, {male, female}, {Arizona, California, Montana, New York}, {short, tall}, {Asian, African-American, Caucasian, Hispanic, Native American, Polynesian}, {straight, curly}, and so on. Some categorical variables are ordinal. The distinction between categorical variables and qualitative variables is a bit blurry. C.f. quantitative variable.

Censoring: When the response variable is the time until an event, subjects not followed long enough for the event to have occurred have their event times censored at the time of last follow-up. This kind of censoring is right censoring. For example, in a follow-up study, patients entering the study during its last year will be followed a maximum of 1 year, so they will have their time until event censored at 1 year or less. Left censoring means that the time to the event is known to be less than some value. In interval censoring, the time is known to be in a specified interval. Most statistical analyses assume that what causes a subject to be censored is independent of what would cause her to have an event. If this is not the case, informative censoring is said to be present. For example, if a subject is pulled off of a drug because of a treatment failure, the censoring time is indirectly reflecting a bad clinical outcome, and the resulting analysis will be biased.

Cohort study: A study in which all subjects meeting the entry criteria are included. Entry criteria are defined at baseline, such as at time of diagnosis or treatment.

Confidence interval (CI): A CI for a parameter is a random interval constructed from data in such a way that the probability that the interval contains the true value of the parameter can be specified before the data are collected. A 95% CI is an estimate of certainty. It is 95% certain that the true value lies within the given range. A narrow CI is good. A CI that spans 1.0 calls into question the validity of the result.

Confounding: When the differences between the treatment and control groups other than the treatment produce differences in response that are not distinguishable from the effect of the treatment, those differences between the groups are said to be confounded with the effect of the treatment (if any). For example, prominent statisticians questioned whether differences between individuals that led some to smoke and others not to (rather than the act of smoking itself) were responsible for the observed difference in the frequencies with which smokers and nonsmokers contract various illnesses. If that were the case, those factors would be confounded with the effect of smoking. Confounding is quite likely to affect observational studies and experiments that are not randomized. Confounding tends to be decreased by randomization.

Continuous variable: A quantitative variable is continuous if its set of possible values is uncountable. Examples include temperature, exact height, and exact age (including parts of a second). In practice, one can never measure a continuous variable to infinite precision, so continuous variables are sometimes approximated by discrete variables. A random variable X is also called continuous if its set of possible values is uncountable, and the chance that it takes any particular value is zero (in symbols, if $P(X = x) = 0$ for every real number x). A random variable is continuous if and only if its cumulative probability distribution function is a continuous function (a function with no jumps).

Correlation coefficient: The correlation coefficient r is a measure of how nearly a scatterplot falls on a straight line. The correlation coefficient is always between −1 and +1. To compute the correlation coefficient of a list of pairs of measurements (X,Y), first transform X and Y individually into standard units. Multiply corresponding elements of the transformed pairs to get a single list of numbers. The correlation coefficient is the mean of that list of products. This page contains a tool that lets you generate bivariate data with any correlation coefficient you want.

Crossover study: A study that compares the results of a two treatment on the same group of patients. The sample size calculated for a crossover study can also be used for a study that compares the value of a variable after treatment with its value before treatment. The standard deviation (SD) of the outcome variable is expressed as either the within-patient SD or the SD of the difference. The former is the SD of repeated observations in the same individual, and the latter is the SD of the difference between two measurements in the same individual.

Cross-sectional study: A study that involves the observation of all of a population or a representative subset at one specific point in time. An example would be to measure cholesterol levels in daily walkers across two age groups, over 40 and under 40, and compare these to cholesterol levels among non-walkers in the same age groups. One can even create subgroups for gender. However, one would not consider past or future cholesterol levels, for these would fall outside the frame. Only cholesterol levels at one point in time would be considered.

Dependent variable: In regression, the variable whose values are supposed to be explained by changes in the other variable (the independent or explanatory variable). Usually one regresses the dependent variable on the independent variable.

Double blind: In a double-blind experiment, neither the subjects nor the people evaluating the subjects know who is in the treatment group and who is in the control group. This mitigates the placebo effect and guards against conscious and unconscious prejudice for or against the treatment on the part of the evaluators.

External validity: A study is externally valid or generalizable if it can produce unbiased inferences regarding a target population (beyond the subjects in the study).

False-negative: Negative test results in a subject who possesses the attribute for which the test is conducted. The labeling of a diseased person as healthy when screening in the detection of disease.

False-positive: Positive test result in a subject who does not possess the attribute for which the test is being conducted. The labeling of a healthy person as diseased when screening in the detection of disease.

Hazard ratio: The ratio of hazard rates at a single time t for two types of subjects. Hazard ratios are in the interval $(0, \infty)$, and they are frequently good ways to summarize the relative effects of two treatments at a specific time $t$. Similar to odds ratios, hazard ratios can apply to any level of outcome probability for the reference group. Note that a hazard ratio is distinct from a risk ratio, the latter being the ratio of two simple probabilities and not the ratio of two rates.

Incidence: The rate of occurrence of new cases of a disease or condition in a population at risk during a given period of time, usually 1 year.

Independent variable: In regression, the variable that is supposed to explain the other; the term is a synonym for *explanatory variable*. Usually one regresses the "dependent variable" on the "independent variable." There is not always a clear choice of the independent variable. The independent variable is usually plotted on the horizontal axis. *Independent* in this context does not mean the same thing as *statistically independent*.

Internal validity: The index and comparison groups are selected and compared in such a manner that the observed differences between them on the dependent variables under study may, apart from sampling error, be attributed only to the hypothesized effect under investigation.

Likelihood ratio (LR): A LR greater than 1 indicates an increased likelihood of disease, and LR less than 1 indicates a decreased likelihood of disease.

The most helpful tests generally have a ratio of less than 0.2 or greater than 5.

Mean: Arithmetic average; the sum of all the values divided by the number of observations. The mean can be heavily influenced by outliers.

Measurement bias: Systematic error arising from inaccurate measurement (or classification) of subjects on the study variables.

Median: The "middle value" of a list. The smallest number such that at least half the numbers in the list are no greater than it. If the list has an odd number of entries, the median is the middle entry in the list after sorting the list into increasing order. If the list has an even number of entries, the median is the smaller of the two middle numbers after sorting. The median can be estimated from a histogram by finding the smallest number such that the area under the histogram to the left of that number is 50%.

Metaanalysis: A type of systematic review that uses rigorous statistical methods to quantitatively synthesize the results of multiple similar studies.

Mode: For lists, the mode is a most common (frequent) value. A list can have more than one mode. For histograms, a mode is a relative maximum ("bump").

Normal distribution: A symmetric, bell-shaped distribution that is most useful for approximating the distribution of statistical estimators. Also called the Gaussian distribution. For a normal distribution, the probability that a measurement will fall within ±1.96 standard deviations of the mean is 0.95.

Number needed to harm: The number of patients who need to receive an intervention instead of the alternative in order for one additional patient to experience an adverse event.

Number needed to treat (NNT): The number of patients who need to receive an intervention instead of the alternative in order for one additional patient to benefit. The NNT is calculated as: 1/ARR. Example: if the ARR (absolute risk reduction) is 4%, the NNT = ¼% = 1/0.04 = 25.

Observational study: A study in which no experimental condition (e.g., treatment) is manipulated by the investigator.

Ordinal variable: A variable whose possible values have a natural order, such as {short, medium, long}, {cold, warm, hot}, or {0, 1, 2, 3, ...}. In contrast, a variable whose possible values are {straight, curly} or {Arizona, California, Montana, New York} would not naturally be ordinal. Arithmetic with the possible values of an ordinal variable does not necessarily make sense, but it does make sense to say that one possible value is larger than another.

P (probability) Value: The probability that a test statistic would be as extreme as or more extreme than observed if the null hypothesis was true. The letter P followed is by the abbreviation n.s. (not significant) or a number is a statement of the probability that the difference observed could have occurred by chance if the groups are really alike. In most biomedical and epidemiologic work, a study result whose probability value is less than 5% ($P < 0.05$) or

1% ($P$ <0.01) is considered sufficiently unlikely to have occurred by chance to justify the designation "statistically significant."

Parallel design: A parallel designed clinical trial compares the results of a treatment on two separate groups of patients. The sample size calculated for a parallel design can be used for any study in which two groups are being compared.

Phase I study: Studies to obtain preliminary information on dosage, absorption, metabolism, and the relationship between toxicity and the dose schedule of treatment.

Phase II study: Studies to determine feasibility and estimate treatment activity and safety in diseases (or, for example, tumor types) for which the treatment appears promising. Generates hypotheses for later testing.

Phase III study: Comparative trial to determine the effectiveness and safety of a new treatment relative to standard therapy. These trials usually represent the most rigorous proof of treatment efficacy (pivotal trials) and are the last stage before product licensing.

Phase IV study: Postmarketing studies of licensed products.

Posttest probability: Probability of disease after a test is performed.

Power: The probability that a clinical trial will have a significant(positive) result, that is, have a $P$ value of less than the specified significance level (usually 5%). This probability is computed under the assumption that the treatment difference or strength of association equals the minimal detectable difference. The power of a test against a specific alternative hypothesis is the chance that the test correctly rejects the null hypothesis when the alternative hypothesis is true. Increases with increasing sample size.

Precision: Degree of absence of random error. Precision can be quantified by the width of a confidence interval and sometimes by a standard deviation of the estimator (standard error). For the confidence intervals, a "margin for error" is computed so that the quoted interval has a certain probability of containing the true value (e.g., population mean difference). By that definition, precision increases linearly as the sample size increases. If one defines precision on the original scale of measurement instead of its square (i.e., if one uses the standard error or width of a confidence interval), precision increases as the square root of the sample size.

Prevalence: The number of people in a population with a specific disease or condition at a given time, usually expressed as a ratio of the number of affected people to the total population.

Prospective study: Study in which the study is first designed and then the subjects are enrolled. Prospective studies are usually characterized by intentional data collection.

Quartiles: The 25th and 75th percentiles and the median. The three values divide variables distributions into four intervals containing equal numbers of observations.

Random error: An error caused by sampling from a group rather than knowing the true value of a quantity such as the mean blood pressure for the entire group (e.g., healthy men older than 80 years of age). One can also speak of random errors in single measurements for individual subjects (e.g., the er).

Randomization: Allocation of individuals to groups, such as for experimental and control regimens, by chance. Within the limits of chance variation, randomization should make the control and experimental groups similar at the start of an investigation.

Randomized controlled trial: An epidemiologic experiment in which subjects in a population are randomly allocated into groups, usually called "study" and "control" groups, to receive or not receive an experimental preventive or therapeutic procedure or intervention.

Recall bias: Systematic error caused by differences in accuracy or completeness of recall to memory of prior events or experiences.

Regression, linear: Linear regression fits a line to a scatterplot in such a way as to minimize the sum of the squares of the residuals. The resulting regression line, together with the standard deviations (SDs) of the two variables or their correlation coefficient, can be a reasonable summary of a scatterplot if the scatterplot is roughly football shaped. In other cases, it is a poor summary. If we are regressing the variable Y on the variable X and if Y is plotted on the vertical axis and X is plotted on the horizontal axis, the regression line passes through the point of averages and has slope equal to the correlation coefficient times the SD of Y divided by the SD of X.

Relative risk (RR): The ratio of the risk of disease or death among the exposed to the risk among the unexposed; this usage is synonymous with risk ratio.

Relative risk reduction (RRR): The percentage difference in risk or outcomes between treatment and control groups. Example: if the mortality rate is 30% in control participants and 20% with treatment, RRR is $(30 - 20)/30 = 33\%$.

Reliability: The degree of stability exhibited when a measurement is repeated under identical conditions. Reliability refers to the degree to which the results obtained by a measurement procedure can be replicated.

Reporting bias: Selective suppression or revealing of information such as past history of sexually transmitted disease.

Response bias: Systematic error caused by a difference in characteristics between those who choose or volunteer to participate in a study and those who do not.

Retrospective study: A research design that is used to test etiologic hypotheses in which inferences about exposure to the putative causal factor(s) are derived from data relating to characteristics of the persons under study or to events or experiences in their past.

ROC (receiver operating characteristic) curve: A plot of sensitivity vs. one minus specificity of all possible dichotomizations of a marker as the cutpoints are varied. The area under the ROC curve is one way to summarize the diagnostic discrimination of a test. The closer this value is to 1, the better the test is at discriminating disease from nondiseased states.

Sample size: The number of patients or experimental units required for the trial.

Sampling bias: Unless the sampling method ensures that all members of the "universe" or reference population have a known chance of inclusion in the sample, bias is possible.

Selection bias: Error caused by systematic differences in characteristics between those who are selected for study and those who are not. Selection bias also invalidates generalizable conclusions from surveys that would include only volunteers from a healthy population.

Sensitivity: Percentage of patients with disease who have a positive test result for the disease in question.

Specificity: Percentage of patients without disease who have a negative test result for the disease in question.

Standard deviation (SD): A measure of the variability (spread) of measurements across subjects. In a normal distribution, the mean $\pm1.96$ SD is expected to cover 95% of the distribution of the measurement. SD is the square root of the variance.

Standard error: The standard deviation (SD) of a statistical estimator. For example, the SD of a mean is called the standard error of the mean, and it equals the SD of individual measurements divided by the square root of the sample size. Standard errors describe the precision of a statistical summary, not the variability across subjects. Standard errors go to zero as the sample size $\rightarrow \infty$.

Survival analysis: A branch of statistics dealing with the analysis of the time until an event such as death. Survival analysis is distinguished by its emphasis on estimating the time course of events and in dealing with censoring.

Systematic review: A type of review article that uses explicit methods to comprehensively analyze and qualitatively synthesize information from multiple studies.

Time to an event: The outcome of the study is a time, such as the time to death, or relapse. Some patients will not have been observed to relapse. These observations are said to be censored.

Type I error: Type of error that occurs when the null hypothesis is rejected erroneously when it is in fact true.

Type II error: Type of error that occurs if the null hypothesis is not rejected when it is in fact false.

Validity, study: The degree to which the inference drawn from a study, especially generalizations extending beyond the study sample, are warranted when account is taken of the study methods, the representativeness of the study sample, and the nature of the population from which it is drawn.

# INDEX

Page numbers followed by *f* or *t* indicate figures or tables respectively.

Lightning Source UK Ltd.
Milton Keynes UK
UKHW020959110721
386985UK00004B/15